ANDTHAT'S WHY
YOU'RE
FAT

Health & Fitness Mistakes
to Stop Making

Lose Fat, Boost Metabolism,
Get the Body You Want NOW!

DR.PHOENYX AUSTIN

And That's Why You're Fat: Health & Fitness Mistakes to Stop Making- Lose Fat, Boost Metabolism & Get the Body You Want NOW (Volume 1) by Phoenyx Austin, M.D.

(Formerly) And That's Why You're Fat: Health & Fitness Mistakes You Don't Know You're Making by Phoenyx Austin, M.D.

Website: drphoenyx.com

Copyright © 2013 by Tracy Austin

ISBN 978-0-9848630-2-0

Printed in the United States of America

Published by Phoenyx Austin

Disclaimer

The ideas, concepts and opinions expressed in *And That's Why You're Fat: Health & Fitness Mistakes to Stop Making*, are solely intended to be used for educational purposes. This book is sold with the understanding that the author and publisher are not rendering medical advice of any kind, nor is the information in this book intended to replace medical advice, or to diagnose, prescribe or treat any disease, condition, illness or injury.

The author and publisher claim no responsibility to any person or entity for any liability, loss, or damage caused or alleged to be caused directly or indirectly as a result of the use, application or interpretation of the material in this book.

Please consult with your doctor before beginning any nutrition or exercise program.

"When you know better, do better." — Maya Angelou

To my best friend, my partner in crime, my inspiration. I love you madly, and always will.

Acknowledgements

If we stand tall, it is because we stand on the shoulders of many ancestors. — African Proverb

I can stand tall as a health and fitness expert, and most importantly, as a human being, because I've been fortunate to cross paths with briliant teachers and mentors who've selflessly shared their wisdom, positivity and love. A deep, heartfelt thank you to my family, my closest friends, and the remarkable colleagues I've come to befriend throughout the years. Last, but definitely not least, thank you to all my fans and readers. As much as this is book is for you, it is also for the little girl in me who believes in following her dreams. Words could never fully express how incredibly awesome it is to wake up every morning and do what I love, while following my passion to make the world a better and fitter place. Thank you all so much for your support. You guys rock!

Table of Contents

WHAT'S UP, DOC?!

Hey guys! I'm Dr. Phoenyx Austin, but you can call me "Doc" for short. Professionally speaking, I'm a Sports Medicine Physician, Certified Fitness Trainer, and #1 Bestselling author of *And That's Why You're Fat: Health & Fitness Mistakes to Stop Making*. Personally speaking, I'm a woman who loves being active, who loves activities like rock climbing, CrossFit, extreme sports, kickboxing, running, and swimming. Oh, and one more thing—I'm also a woman whose home is practically littered with sporting gear and fitness magazines. So yeah, I live and breathe fitness and I'm an all-around fitness junkie.

And now that we've been formally introduced, I want to share a story about my professional journey as a health and fitness expert, as well as my personal journey to becoming a healthier individual. This way, by taking a brief trip down memory lane, you can get an even better understanding of me, my passion for fitness, and why I wrote this book.

How did it all start for me, and how did I get here?

Well, first off let me say that in my humble opinion, exercise and nutrition are the greatest forms of medicine—hands down! Exercise and nutrition are two highly effective tools that I regularly use to help others improve their level of fitness, as well as their lives in general. Exercise and nutrition are also two tools that I've used personally to build an awesome career and life for myself. I absolutely love what I do, and I love the fact that I get to positively impact people's lives on a daily basis.

I must say that in a philosophical kind of way, I believe fitness is just a metaphor for life in general. Simply put, I have no doubt that if you can achieve big things *inside* the gym you can most certainly achieve big things *outside*. So it's no wonder that I absolutely love sharing fitness advice for people who want to get in shape, because in my heart of hearts I know that those same people will ultimately take the principles I've shared with them and use those very same principles to not just improve their bodies, but to better themselves as individuals overall. No doubt, getting in shape is an infectious thing and a sort of gateway drug. It boosts confidence, and the confidence spills over into other parts of one's life. I see it all the time with my clients and everyday people. These people transform their bodies *and* they also transform their minds at the same time without even realizing it. The woman with low self-esteem becomes self-assured and confident. The shy guy becomes more outspoken, commanding more respect from his peers. Taking control of their bodies, for many people, allows them to ultimately take control of their lives.

"FAT!" DID YOU REALLY JUST CALL PEOPLE FAT?!?

When brainstorming titles for this book, I wanted something that was real, that was down to earth, that was non-PC, and that spoke to people across the board. I wanted something that would roll off the tongue and sear itself into the brain. Hence, *And That's Why You're Fat* was born. And yes, the title of my book may even be a little provocative. I realize that some people will get a good chuckle from my title, while some people might get offended. To the amused, hey, I'm laughing along with you. And to those I may have offended, what can I say other than I can refer you to an excellent proctologist to help you remove the stick from your butt.

Look, at the end of the day, this book isn't meant to upset or "fat shame" anyone. It's meant to be educational and engaging. Even more important, it's meant to inspire. I want you to really enjoy reading this book and I want you to learn—A LOT! There's a ton of good stuff here that I want you to absorb. So please take all the information contained in my book and use it to achieve your fitness goals, whatever they may be.

Because let me tell you, I absolutely relish the smile on a client's face when she reports that she's lost five pounds in the past month. And I also get a kick out of the way a male client puffs out his chest like a peacock when he talks about increasing his personal best on the bench press. I love to see good people win in the gym and at life. It totally turns me on. It's my aphrodisiac. I sincerely want you to get healthy, fit and happy. When you're healthy, fit and happy, I get happy too. See, everybody wins!

THIS ISN'T AS HARD AS IT SEEMS—TRUST ME!

Whenever I write, I always like to get into the heads of my readers so I can better understand their needs. In many ways, this is the book I wish I had when I started "formally" learning about fitness several years ago—back when I was wading through a lot of bad advice and blatant misinformation, and just trying to get down to the basic truth of what it really means to eat healthy and exercise for specific results like losing fat, building muscle or building endurance.

There were times during those early days in my fitness education that I also got frustrated, but I never let up because I'm just so passionate about this topic and what I do. I actually viewed all of the obstacles I faced as a challenge of sorts and a test of my will to learn and ultimately become an outstanding fitness expert. And let me tell you something about myself: I'll never back down from a challenge of my mental, intellectual and physical strength.

Believe me when I say that I totally empathize with all of you fitness newbies that get frustrated by all the contradictory and confusing fitness information floating around. It seems like every month you're running across some new fitness article in a popular print or online magazine that seemingly contradicts a similar fitness article that you just read last month. All of this contradictory advice can become intolerable and I totally get why people get fed up, throw up their hands and say, "To hell with it all! I'll just stay fat and out of shape!

If this sounds all too familiar, take a deep sigh of relief because those days are over. You'll no longer feel confused or frustrated. When I wrote this book, I kept all of the above in mind. I kept you, the reader, in mind. I sincerely want you to have the healthiest and best body you can achieve. And trust me when I say that getting educated about fitness, exercise and nutrition is not difficult or confusing. You just need an excellent teacher (ME!) who will present the facts to you in an objective way that's easy to absorb and implement.

THE IMPORTANCE OF PERSONAL RESPONSIBILITY (MY PART)

Now not too long ago I was a medical student—a bright-eyed, bushy-tailed and eager doctor-to-be ready to spread the health and wellness gospel. Yet ironically enough, during that very important time in my professional path to becoming a full-fledged *M.D.*, I gradually found myself losing touch with who I was as an individual, as well as with my passions and my core values. What do I mean by all that? Well, basically, I slowly began not following the same advice I was dishing out to others in regards to health and wellness. And as more and more time went on in my medical education, there was a growing and clear disconnect between what I was practicing and what I was preaching.

What was causing this disconnect?

Well, I could point to a few reasons, one of the biggest being that medical training is incredibly demanding and oftentimes requires functioning under high stress with little time for even the basic necessities—like sleep. So like most medical students, I adapted to the demands of school and training by overindulging in a few not-so-healthy habits, like downing tons of sugary sweet caffeinated drinks to keep me energized, eating obscene amounts of quick-'n'-easy carb-ilicious fast foods, and barely getting any exercise. And what was the end result of my brilliant approach to life? Exactly what you'd expect. I got fat! At my heaviest, I was lugging around 155 pounds on my small 5'2" frame.

To camouflage my weight, I started to hide behind hospital scrubs and my white coat. I was also frequently tired and just felt sluggish and very *blah* in general. It was not a good look at all. As time went on, I began to grow very disenchanted with my physical appearance, and despite the fact that I earned a professional title that instantaneously garnered so much respect (*paging Dr. Phoenyx!*), I usually felt very insecure about my appearance and myself overall as a person. To top it all off, I kinda started to feel like a major hypocrite (I'll explain more about that below).

All my life I'd been a very active and a very health-conscious person. Growing up, I was a huge tomboy (*and I still very much am!*). I loved sports, being outdoors, and hitting the gym. But now, as a physician in training, I barely had the energy to work out, and taking care of my body seemed to take a constant backseat to all of my other professional responsibilities. *Not quite the lifestyle I pictured for myself as a young and budding doc who went into the health profession because she actually believed in the importance of things like health, fitness and wellness.*

So despite all my actions to the contrary, I can assure you that deep down inside I absolutely did not want to be the physician that was overweight, barely able to jog a mile, self-medicating with cheese puffs, and all the while telling patients how *they* needed to take care of themselves and get in shape. That's definitely not the doc I signed up to be. On top of that, I'm a woman who takes pride in her body. And I'll be frank, I like to look good—damn good, in fact! I mean seriously, what woman doesn't?!

The thing many people don't realize about being a doctor is that the whole lifestyle is set up with numerous landmines that make it pretty darn easy for doctors to get out of shape and become unhealthy ourselves. Many medical students and young doctors are overworked and stressed out. Because of this fact, many of my colleagues and docs-in-training end up making poor lifestyle choices. But that's a whole other topic in itself. Suffice it to say that the path to becoming a doctor is a great test not only of intelligence, but also of physical and emotional resolve. So I have immense respect for my fellow physicians who bust their butts every day to make this world a healthier place.

That said, my thoughts are also that if you've chosen to become a health professional—doctor or otherwise, overworked or not—you should not just focus on being the "messenger" of good health. You owe yourself much more than that. **It's also about taking personal**

responsibility. You owe it to yourself to take care of yourself. Moreover, speaking as a health and fitness professional, my thoughts are that my fellow colleagues should not just be talking the talk—we should be walking the walk. Health and fitness professionals should be an inspiration to others, not just through our words, but also through our physical appearance. That's my personal and professional opinion. And that's what motivates me. Because I want to be fit and healthy myself. Because I truly believe in the professional oath I took as a physician, and because I want to inspire others.

Now, I do want you to understand that I'm not telling you all this to put my overweight colleagues in the hot seat. Rather, I'm telling you this to illustrate the very important point that doctors are human just like everyone else. Doctors are human and we have flaws. Many doctors struggle with weight issues just like the average person. I know I sure did. I've had my battles with the bulge and with emotional eating, and I still have some struggles to this day. I also made a ton of mistakes with how I approached my diet and exercise, but I love to learn and I'm passionate about fitness, so I eagerly sought out ways to educate myself until I got it right. Getting to where I am today involved reading tons of books and articles and talking with as many fitness and nutrition experts as I could.

Moreover, my journey from *fat* to *fit* involved a lot of "non-classroom" education and even a bit of experimentation on my own body. Unbeknownst to many people, nutrition and exercise courses are not part of the standard medical school curriculum. So when it came to learning about fitness, exercise and nutrition, sometimes it felt like I was literally steering my ship without a compass. In the end, I've put in a lot of leg work into expanding my knowledge base so I could become a well-rounded health and fitness professional. Why? Because I believe that as individuals we should constantly be in a state of seeking knowledge and truth so we can continue to grow and evolve into better versions of ourselves.

The knowledge I've gained from being both a medical doctor and a certified personal trainer means that I come with two distinct, yet very interrelated skill sets. As a physician, I have a medical background and in-depth knowledge about topics like anatomy, biology and biochemistry. As a fitness trainer, I have in-depth knowledge about topics like exercise physiology, nutrition, and even psychology. This book represents the merging of my two skill sets and professional expertise. I must say that it's pretty cool to walk the line between doctor and trainer, because I see fitness from many angles and perspectives that the average doctor and even the average trainer may not see.

Still, I give credit where credit is due, and my growth as a health and fitness professional is also the result of excellent teachers. I didn't get to where I am all by myself. Furthermore, I know for a fact that it's not just my book smarts and professional titles that make me a credible expert on health and fitness. It's one thing to spout off a bunch of "facts" about diet, exercise, health and nutrition. But it's a whole other thing to be able to effectively communicate with the average person, as well as put your money where your mouth is and show people what is possible with your own body. So I know that it's not just my degrees and book smarts that make me credible; it's also my success with clients, as well as my own personal success with losing weight, that has made me a "health and fitness expert."

THE IMPORTANCE OF PERSONAL RESPONSIBILITY (YOUR PART)

Let me say it now so it will be forever known where I stand regarding you and your body: *You are 100 percent responsible for your own health.*

Truth be told, it's not your doctor's (or anyone else's) job to nag you about your health or convince you to lose weight. And I know it's a bit of a rhetorical question, but I still have to ask: Why do some of us adults carry this absurd notion that it's anyone else's responsibility but our own to take care of ourselves?

Now, I'm going to spend a bit of time on my "personal responsibility" soapbox because this point sorely needs to emphasized—especially in this day and age when far too many people don't like to accept personal responsibility. Nowadays, people like to go in on health professionals, especially doctors. Blaming my fellow colleagues for not doing enough to totally cure the very same health problems many of these people bring on themselves—which really grinds my gears because it's not your doctor's job to make you care about your health or take care of yourself. Once again, you are responsible for your health. Period. Full stop.

Furthermore, it is my firm belief that **the one and only reason most people don't succeed with losing weight and getting in shape is because they haven't had enough personal reason to do so.**

More than 36 percent of Americans are now considered obese, according to the U.S. Centers for Disease Control and Prevention. In addition to that, 34 percent are considered overweight. Every day, people are getting sick and dying from obesity-related diseases in record numbers.

That's so crazy and so sad to me. Just think about it: We are a nation that's literally killing itself with crap food and lack of exercise. How does that sit with you?

Look, being fat sucks. Study after study shows that it sucks. But too many people think it's "no big deal" to be fat and on eight different types of medications. And sadly enough, I've also found that some people have a tendency to find a level of comfort in discomfort and dysfunction. They think: *Hey, diabetes is no big deal. I'll just get on some insulin. My insurance is covering it. It's all good!* Clearly these people just haven't had a hot enough fire lit under their butts.

Let me tell you something: Getting sick is expensive, especially if you don't have good health insurance. Diabetes is expensive. Heart attacks are expensive. Strokes are expensive. Medications, ambulance rides and hospitalizations are expensive. And it can get even worse as you get older. When most of us are in our 20s and 30s and cruising through life with a sort of "invincibility complex," it never dawns on us that we may get really sick and not be able to afford home health care or medications because something like a stroke has left us unable to live independently. Trust and believe, the choices you are making now are an investment in your life later down the road—whether the investment is good or bad is up to you. Invest wisely.

LIVING IN A WARZONE

It may come as a shock to some, but the diseases that the vast majority of us are dying from today were nonexistent to our ancestors. Cavemen weren't dropping dead from diabetes, heart disease or cancer. These diseases are a direct result of the unhealthy lifestyles we lead and the horrendous way we treat our bodies. These diseases are consequences of our own making. They are a direct result of bad investments and of being fat and unhealthy.

Guys, today we are living in a warzone. Every day we are being heavily marketed to and bombarded with legal substances (like junk food) that make us sick. And if you are not willing to arm yourself with knowledge so you can take control of your life and your health, your body and physique will suffer. So wake up! This is not a game! It really is a warzone out there. If you choose to remain ignorant of this fact, you will be taken out—be it quickly or slowly.

I know all of the above can sound a bit scary, but being fat, sick and unhealthy never has to be anyone's fate. Obesity and obesity-related illnesses can be totally avoided, reversed and cured. For all of you reading this book, no matter your previous struggles and frustrations, I want you to know that you can lose the weight and you can get in shape.

I truly want to help you achieve your goal of becoming slimmer, stronger, and yes—sexier! But before we can even come anywhere near to accomplishing those goals, you'll first need to accept total responsibility for your health and be 100 percent ready to do what needs to be done to get you where you want to go.

"SIMPLE AND SMART" DOES THE TRICK

I hope I didn't go in too hard on you guys in the last section. I just want to hammer home the importance of taking control of your health in order to have an outstanding quality of life.

And outside of accepting personal responsibility, another huge problem that's preventing many of you from reaching your fitness goals is a lack of education: Lack of education about nutrition and lack of education about exercise. For example, many people have no clue how to read a food label. And many people don't even know what a kettlebell is.

Now on a positive note, I've found that people are indeed hungry for fitness education. They really do want to learn how to pick healthier foods and get in shape. They just don't want things to be overly confusing and contradictory, and I totally get that. Yeah, I'm a pretty smart cookie and I've got more degrees and certifications than you can shake a stick at. But I'll be honest, I hate when fitness information (or information in general) is presented in a way that's pompous, exceedingly verbose and overly complex. I like to keep things simple and to the point. Things that are overly and unnecessarily complex just frustrate me and make my head hurt. Oftentimes, less is indeed more, and that's why I prefer breaking down fitness into the most basic terms, because that's how most people are going to be able to fully digest the information and put it to good use. Simple and smart really does the trick.

That understood, I want to also put it out there that *simple* doesn't always equal *smart*. For example, a simple way to lose weight is just to starve yourself. Eat nothing and you'll lose pounds in no time! But as I'm sure most of you already know (or will soon learn), simply starving yourself isn't very smart. So my overall point here is that my approach to fitness is both simple and smart. I will keep things simple, to the point and easy to follow. As far as this being a "smart" fitness book, I must now inform you that I will delve a bit into "science-y" topics like hormones and nutrition. But rest assured, nothing will be over your head. Basically, I'll be lightly delving into a few of these important "science-y" topics and concepts because it will allow people to start connecting the dots that they didn't connect before. In my opinion, lightly delving into these "science-y" topics will help speed up reader comprehension and arrival at the coveted "aha" fitness moment—that beautiful moment the little light bulb goes on over people's heads and they joyfully exclaim:

So that's why I couldn't lose weight!

In addition to wanting to help you connect all the fitness dots, I also have to admit that I couldn't just totally leave out the more "science-y" stuff because I do enjoy talking about it. Yeah, yeah, I'm a big ol' nerd. I really get turned on by this stuff! And I thoroughly enjoy sharing any information I can with people who are eager to learn about fitness too.

Another thing that turns me on about fitness (and life in general) is how far we've advanced technologically as a society. We have evolved to the point where information is literally at our fingertips. Just hop on sites like Google and YouTube and you can find an abundance of information on just about any topic, including fitness and health. It's really astounding and remarkable when you stop to think about it. Granted, there's also a ton of misinformation floating around. But by and large, I think this is an incredible age we live in, with such easy access to information. There really isn't any fitness- or health-related question that you can't find the answer to if you're willing to do a little research on your PC, laptop, tablet or cell phone.

And it doesn't stop there. Within the arena of exercise and sports science, we have incredibly cool gadgets like heart rate monitors, biofeedback machines and fitness apps that can help anyone control, track and have lots of fun with their fitness journey. Also, you've got state-of-the-art gyms with every piece of exercise equipment imaginable. Heck, you don't even need to go to the gym if you want to get in shape. You can buy all the exercise equipment you need on Amazon, have it shipped to your house, and build your own personal gym. Or you can just get in front of your 50-inch plasma TV and throw in a workout DVD or exercise to your Wii.

The avenues to get in shape really are endless, and I tell people all the time that we live in an awesome time in regards to health and fitness. With access to all this super-cool technology to inform us, work us out and even entertain us while we exercise, in this day and age there is absolutely no reason why anyone should feel "bored" working out or have a significantly hard time getting in shape.

THE BOOK BREAKDOWN

As mentioned earlier, this book is going to be a simple and smart guide to common health and fitness mistakes. Overall, these health and fitness mistakes will pertain to weight loss—or more specifically, fat loss. Yes, there is a distinct difference between losing weight and losing fat. Losing fat results in your body becoming slimmer, stronger and sexier. On the other hand, just losing weight often results in you seeing lower numbers on the bathroom scale while becoming "softer" and "weaker." Gone are the days of super-skinny models with no curves or muscular definition. Most women don't want to look like that. Most women want a slim, toned body, with nice flat abs and a tight, curvy booty. The way to get that look is with fat loss (not just weight loss). *And That's Why You're Fat* is about losing fat, building lean muscle, boosting your metabolism and getting the body you want. So make sure you follow the advice in my book if your goal is to have a slimmer, stronger and sexier body.

In this book, I'm going to address a number of fitness mistakes and fitness myths in a fun, straightforward and educational manner. I'm going to give you the "fitness facts" and teach you how to approach your training and nutrition in a smarter way. Also, you don't necessarily have to read this book in order, so feel free to scan the Table of Contents and jump to whatever sparks your interest the most.

Without a doubt, health, fitness and nutrition myths are as pervasive and as persistent as a post-apocalyptic New York City cockroach. Everywhere you turn, you're almost guaranteed to find folks spouting off fitness myths like the ones you've just read above. Maybe you, yourself, have heard a few of these "nuggets of fitness wisdom" and wondered whether they were fact or fiction.

Here's a little taste of what's to come in the later pages of this book:

> **You say**: Eating late will make you fat.
>
> **I say**: BZZZT – WRONG!
>
> **You say**: Lifting heavy weights will make a woman look like a Dallas Cowboys linebacker in heels.
>
> **I say:** BZZZT – WRONG!
>
> **You say**: Doing a hundred crunches a day will give you a six-pack.
>
> **I say:** BZZZT – WRONG!

This is all to say that I want to help you expand your exercise and nutrition knowledge, broaden your mind, and become fitness-savvy! By the end of this book, you'll finally get the answers to your most burning health and fitness questions, and you'll ultimately learn things about your body and the physiology of weight loss and muscle growth that many people will never know. You'll also gain an advanced level of understanding of how to burn body fat easily, build lean muscle effectively, boost metabolism, feel better overall, and get the body you want easier, faster and more enjoyably than ever before!

Oh, and one more thing. Just a quick heads-up to any fellas who may have picked up this book. Because I tend to work with and focus on women, I have a tendency to naturally reference women and depict scenarios with women, so you will hear me primarily addressing women in this book. That's not to say that the fitness and health information I'm sharing does not apply to men, because it absolutely does! Yes, there are key differences between men and women, but rest assured that the core information and principles of this book are still the same regardless of gender.

6 STEPS TO GETTING THE BODY YOU WANT

Through my career, I've helped countless people get in the best shape of their lives, and all of these people, no matter their initial fitness level, age or background, always did six key things that enabled them to be successful. Before we get deeper into this book, I want you to take the time to read through these six steps. Slacking off on *just one* of these steps could be the very thing that keeps you from getting the body you want.

1. Be an eager student.

Look at this book as a manual on how your body works. If you want to know all the right buttons to push to burn fat, build muscle, and get the hot body you want, then you will need to thoroughly read this manual. It's really no different from when you buy a new gadget or toy. The gadget comes with directions, but a good portion of you will want to skim through the manual or skip reading it all together. You'll just throw in some batteries, start pressing random buttons and see if you can figure things out along the way.

In this day and age, far too many people don't want to take the time to read and learn about their body. That is so crazy to me! You've been blessed with this incredible machine (your body) and you don't want to learn how all the parts work?! Come on!

I can say with absolute certainty that most of you reading this book don't fully understand how your body works. You've also been fed a lot of misinformation and myths about fitness.

I'm clearly an expert in my field, and even I need to keep learning about nutrition, fitness and exercise science because research is constantly being conducted and new things are always being discovered. My point is, no matter how much you *think* you already know about fitness, you must be eager to learn more. Don't be the guy or gal that skips reading the manual. Be smart. Be eager to learn. Be an eager student. That is the only way you'll keep growing and advancing toward your best body.

2. Be ready to work.

If you're hungry for a straightforward and effective approach to fitness, then this book is for you! For those of you who are looking for someone to feed you a bunch of ridiculous BS like, "Sure, you can eat crap six days a week and lose 20 pounds in two days," this book is definitely not for you. Anyone who wants results without real work should just put this book down now, or better yet, give it to someone else who's really ready to learn. This is not a game to me. I am passionate about my area of expertise, and I'll only work with people who are realistic and willing to put in hard work to better themselves. That said, is it possible to lose a considerable amount of weight in a short period of time? Absolutely! I've had clients drop eight to 10 pounds in the first two weeks of my nutritional protocols. But that kind of weight loss will only come with work and sacrifice.

Always think of the end result when you're making sacrifices. Keeping the end result in mind will push you to do what needs to be done. Remember, in fitness and in life, you don't get something for nothing. So the next time you head to the gym, realize that you are on a mission. Like I tell all my clients: Don't show up *just* to show up. Show up to put in work because you want specific results.

3. Don't be afraid to experiment.

Though I emphasize the importance of thoroughly reading your body's "manual," there will also come a point when you'll have to stop *learning* about fitness and just start *doing it.* It's like when people go to school and acquire a ton of book knowledge about a particular subject, but then they go into the real world and have a hard time reaching the level of success they want because they realize that the real world doesn't always follow a textbook.

While you definitely should have a solid foundation of fitness knowledge, I don't want you to become so bogged down with the "facts" that you're afraid to try something different. Case in point: Just look to the biographies of some of the most successful and revered individuals in the fitness game—icons like Jack LaLanne and Arnold Schwarzenegger, and many, many others. These guys came up in a time when the fitness frontier was still very much uncharted territory. But did they let a lack of scientific studies or an abundance of skeptics stop them from trying new things? Absolutely not! And you know what, through their willingness to experiment and push boundaries, these icons helped advance the entire profession. These icons also ended up educating the "experts," and they continue to inspire many generations of fitness experts to come.

So if after reading this book, you think there's a more efficient way to do something, test your theory and see if it works. Though I stand by my words 100 percent, I still don't expect you to take everything I write in this book as gospel. Heck, I don't even listen to everything doctors and trainers say!

This is all to say that overall, while I do strongly advise and encourage you to learn the foundations of fitness, I still want you be an independent and critical thinker. So if you want to experiment and take things a bit further, do it. That's the only way you'll ever know if your theory works, so don't be afraid to try new things. Fact is, the human body is not cut and dry. Two plus two does not always equal four. Sometimes two plus two can actually equal six! And when you take the time to start unraveling the complexities of the human body, that's when things can start to get really fun and fascinating.

4. Think like an athlete, train like an athlete.

Most of us look at the bodies of athletes in awe. *Wow! Her abs are to die for! Wow! His biceps are huge!* We wish we could have their physiques, and the truth many of us hide from is that we all could have great bodies like that if we chose to not shortchange ourselves.

The two key factors separating athletes from average folk are their level of commitment and their intensity. Simply put, athletes don't think or train like average people. Take, for example, the 80/20 rule. I'm sure many of you have heard of the 80/20 food rule, which states that it's OK to eat healthy 80 percent of the time, while allowing yourself the indulgences of junk food 20 percent of the time. The average person loves this 80/20 food rule concept. But ask elite athletes their thoughts on the 80/20 rule, and they'd instinctively look at you like you're crazy. To an elite athlete—at least the one who wants to be at the top of his or her game—the 80/20 food rule can be career suicide, and is just another way of conceding to yourself that you're happy with being in 2nd place or 2nd best. And I'll tell you right now, if you hear elite athletes telling you they're cool with 2nd best, they are lying to you and themselves. Trust and believe, athletes want to win. They want the glory. They want to be number one.

In fact, when athletes train, they follow a more stringent diet, often a 90/10 food rule or stricter, depending on their training goals. I've even worked with some athletes that never had a cheat meal while training weeks on end for an important event. This is not to say that "cheat meals" are inherently "evil" and serve no purpose other than to satisfy cravings of the "weak-willed." And for the athletes that do have cheat meals, often they're having them not for the reasons that the average person has a cheat meal. Unbeknownst to many people, cheat meals, when strategically planned and implemented, are actually a very effective tool for boosting metabolism and fat loss.

The point I want to make here is that top athletes understand that it takes a strict level of dedication and sacrifice to reach their goals. Furthermore, they don't just eat for pleasure; they eat for a specific purpose—to prime their body for performance. Athletes don't question why they have to work hard. They don't make excuses. They don't whine about things. They just do what they have to do to be the best and win. And that's how you need to start thinking and acting.

In a nutshell, my thoughts are this: *You should always think of yourself as an athlete.* I don't care if you're 25 or 52 years old—you are an athlete. Get in that mindset. Covet your body. Push yourself a little harder. Especially you guys that are drastically overweight, obese, and maybe even suffering from conditions like diabetes and high blood pressure. Now is the time to quit "skating by" on things like the 80/20 rule. Push yourself. Athletes that need to drastically improve their performance and health don't cheat on their diets 20 percent of the time.

In addition to stepping up adherence to your diet, part of being an athlete also requires stepping up your exercise intensity. I see some of you guys in the gym, talking on your cell phones while you're on the treadmill. Reading a magazine while you're on the elliptical. Taking up space on the weight machine while you fiddle with your MP3 player or cellphone. And there is nothing that chaps my rear end more than two people sitting on weight machines side by side talking! Taking up not one machine, but two!

Oh, no they didn't!

Look, if you can multitask that much when you're exercising, it means you're not going hard enough. Put away the distractions and get to work! Lack of intensity is what separates the average from the athlete. Remember, you are not average. You are an athlete. So if you want the body of an athlete, think like it and act like it!

5. Plan for success.

As the saying goes, *Failing to plan is planning to fail.* No way around it, to be successful in life you will need to become a meticulous planner. I'm not saying you'll need to be OCD, but you will need to plan and journal. In regards to your fitness journey, you will need to do things like make a workout schedule and create a weekly/monthly meal plan or food journal. This is the only surefire way to success. Interestingly enough, many of the people that complain about "not having enough time to exercise" or "not having enough time to cook" are oftentimes falling victim to poor planning and prioritization. Stop making yourself a victim of circumstance due to poor planning. When you are in control of your life, you will be in control of your body.

6. Have fun!

Last of all, I want you to do one more thing—have fun! What good is this journey and life if you can't look back on the entire experience with fond memories? Don't get so caught up in the "goal" of hitting a certain weight or attaining your "dream body" that you forget to have fun getting there. Try new activities, meet new people, make friends and create wonderful memories for yourself. Have fun! Having fun is what will keep you motivated to stay fit for life. And having fun makes all this, even the struggles and sacrifice, worthwhile. Funny thing is, I get emails and people drop in on my social media pages all the time to ask me how I stay motivated to eat healthy and exercise. The simple answer is that all of this, all I do, is just part of who I am. I'm not trying to do something I don't inherently enjoy, and I'm having tons of fun staying active, learning new things and meeting interesting people. So ultimately, I stay motivated and committed for one simple fact: Because I love this stuff!

So from here on out, you are the master of your fate. The formula to your success is going to be very simple and breaks down like this: :

I teach + You learn = You get the body you want.

It's a very simple formula and it works 100 percent of the time. I promise you, everything will fall into place if we can stick to this formula. You will lose the weight, you will get in the best shape of your life, and you will feel awesome! And I will feel awesome for you!

The "New You" Pledge

I like pledges and positive daily affirmations. So I wanted to include this fitness pledge. This pledge is your commitment to a "New You," and I'd love for you to take this pledge with me.

- I will love my body, and know that I can be healthy and fit at any age.

- I will be thankful every day, rejoicing in the fact that each new day is a gift to pursue my fitness goals.

- I will love myself when I am strong, and I will be kind to myself when I am weak.

- I will not use dieting as a temporary fix, but rather, will commit to healthy eating as a permanent lifestyle change.

- I will drink more water and enjoy the benefits it brings to my body and overall health.

- I will work hard, celebrate my successes, and routinely reward myself for my determination and willpower.

- I will not beat myself up when I slip up, which I know will happen because I'm human.

- I will never be too prideful or ashamed to ask for help when I'm struggling.

- I will enjoy my fitness journey, have lots of fun along the way, try new activities and find a way to be active every day.

- I will support my fellow brothers and sisters who are also working hard to achieve their fitness goals.

- I will encourage and be an inspiration to anyone who wants to lead a healthier life.

Alrighty! Now that we have all that out of the way, let's get to the good stuff!

MISTAKE 1
I DON'T HAVE TIME TO EAT HEALTHY AND EXERCISE

YOU SAY: I don't have time to eat healthy and exercise.

I SAY: According to the American Council on Exercise, "not having enough time" is the most common excuse people give or not exercising. But did I really need the American Council on Exercise to tell me that? No, not really.

As a doctor and personal trainer, I often get a double whammy of excuses from people on why they a) don't have time to exercise, or b) don't have enough time, money or whatever to eat healthier foods. And though I can definitely empathize with the fact that we're *all* extremely busy these days running from one obligation to the next, I refuse to get with any of those "I don't have time" excuses.

Yes, I've been accused of having a bit of a drill sergeant mentality when it comes to fitness, and let me explain why. Assuming you're blessed enough to get a full eight hours of sleep every night, that leaves 112 waking hours available to you throughout the week. Now let's assume you're working a 9-to-5. That means we'll have to subtract 40 from 112, which leaves approximately 72 hours at your disposal to squeeze in exercise and meal planning.

Now that I've broken down the numbers, would any of you be willing to put your hand on a Bible and swear that you *really* don't have the "time" in those 72 hours each week to exercise and cook a healthy meal?

It's simple numbers and planning, guys. So maybe you can now see why I just can't accept the "not enough time" defense.

The real issue here boils down to priorities. Simply put: You make time for the things that are important to you, the activities that you really care about. So now let me ask, *How important is your body and your health to you?*

If it's important to you, you'll make the time to take care of yourself. Period. No debate. End of discussion.

And even if you don't inherently "love" exercise, it's important that you get started with some sort of physical activity, even if it's just walking a couple of miles a day. That said, I believe 100-percent that for most people who say they "don't like exercise," it's really an issue of just not being introduced to the *right* physical activities.

Growing up, I used to hate when adults would say general things like, *"In life you have to do things you don't like to do. That's life."* I think that's terrible advice to just throw out willy-nilly every time someone complains about not liking something. Look, I know from personal experience that life is about sacrifice and not every day will be peaches and cream and cotton candy clouds. But even still, I sure don't think life in general, or the pursuit of a fit body, needs to suck overall and be an exercise in self-flagellation. Forget that! Overall, I think life and fitness should be fun. Lots of fun! And if it isn't fun, something is definitely wrong and needs a bit of modification.

So if you've found that you just hate exercising, have always hated exercise and can't bear the thought of exercise, well maybe I'd say it's high time you start looking at getting out of your bubble and start trying new activities that better jive with your temperament and personality.

For example, I had a client who "hated" working out—I mean absolutely hated it! She once told me she'd rather slide down a barbed wire banister into a tub of alcohol than exercise. Before we star working together, she primarily worked out at home alone with boring, generic fitness DVDs. Then I introduced her to rock climbing and Spinning. Now she's a certifiable fitness junkie. Every time I talk to her, she's finding a new rock to climb or raving about her last Spin class. And because she loves these activities so much and does them regularly, she's lost a ton of weight and is now in fantastic shape. In retrospect, her weight loss was just a byproduct of being more active through physical activities she loves. And I think this is the case for everyone who claims that they "hate" exercise. I truly believe that once you find an activity that gets you amped and makes you feel good, you'll be hooked and the positive results will flow from there.

One more thing. For other people who say they "hate exercise," it might not be that you "hate exercise," but rather that you may just be more of an introvert who doesn't like exercising with other people. There are many people like this who join gyms everyday but ironically never use their gym memberships because they feel uncomfortable in the more extroverted atmosphere. I can relate to this because I'm an introvert, and though I still love going to the gym and participating in group classes, I also find that I can really get in my fitness zone when I'm doing solitary activities like taking long walks, running long distances, hiking, swimming or even just working out at home.

When it comes to eating healthy, it's not uncommon for people to say that dieting and eating healthy just plain sucks. If you're one of those people who hates eating "healthy" foods because you think healthy foods taste terrible, maybe it's because you follow terrible (and typical) dieting advice and just need to get better educated about nutrition and food options. With regard to food and nutrition, I am a proponent of low-carb diets, particularly the Ketogenic Diet. Low-carb diets like the Ketogenic Diet are far from restrictive and are not like traditional, low-calorie, low-fat diets. In fact, I think of low-carb as a nutritional lifestyle more than a diet because it's something that can be followed for life rather than temporarily—unlike the "traditional diet." Furthermore, I believe going low-carb makes dieting a lot easier, more sustainable and more pleasurable because it expands your culinary repertoire. And let me tell you, I have yet to find one single person who's told me that they hate eating things like deviled eggs, bacon and eggs, prosciutto-wrapped asparagus spears, chicken Caesar salad, and Greek yogurt with dark chocolate bits—which, incidentally, are very healthy foods and typical low-carb meal options. Personally, I'd rather eat things like that and not the "typical" foods dieters choose to dine on like watery skim milk, plain oatmeal, dry rice cakes and teeny-tiny 100-calorie snack packs. So if you've found yourself "hating" the food options on your diet, I'd strongly advise that you look into low-carb and the Ketogenic Diet, or Keto Diet for short.

OK, by now I'm sure you're all amped and you've decided to start getting to work on your fitness and nutrition plan. Congrats to you! But first I must emphasize something else regarding exercise: When it comes to exercise, don't just say you're going to work out—strategically plan things out. Make a fitness calendar that clearly highlights what exactly you're going to be doing, when you're going to do it, and for how long. And make it simple for yourself. If you want a more varied fitness calendar that rotates days of running, strength training, boot camp class, or whatever, then schedule that. If you just want to just focus on doing your Insanity DVDs, then only schedule that. And for those of you who are really pressed for time, keep in mind that when workouts are planned strategically, getting in shape and staying in shape will not take a lot of time. Gone are the long, drawn-out days in the gym. Exercise science has shown that fitness protocols like 20-minute circuit training sessions and 20-minute high-intensity interval training (HIIT) sessions are excellent for burning calories and building lean muscle mass. Also, simple exercises, like jumping rope and kettlebell workouts, can torch major calories in shorter periods of time.

Fun Fact: One minute of kettlebell training can burn 20 calories!

When it comes down to it, you just need to get stealth about your fitness. Plan and attack! Remember, it's not just about *having* a calendar. It's about having a calendar that you **actually follow and stick to.** Ultimately, with a simple, clear plan of action, your workout sessions will flow better and you'll be more likely to stick to your schedule.

If lack of motivation is something you struggle with when it comes time to exercise, try getting someone else involved to provide that extra push to getting you going. Hire a personal trainer. Ask a friend to be your workout buddy. Whatever option or options you choose, having this sense of accountability is a great way to force yourself to get up and moving.

Another motivational tactic I highly recommend to everyone is rewarding yourself with mini-prizes, one for each step accomplished on the way to your overall fitness goal. Oftentimes people don't do this and instead just plan one big *shebang*, like a cruise or a trip to Vegas, once they meet their overall fitness goal. But sometimes having a reward too far in the future can tempt people to slack off or even become discouraged if they can't fully visualize the finish line. For example, instead of giving yourself one big, solitary reward after dropping the total 30 pounds you've been working to lose, you can instead reward yourself every time you drop five pounds. The gifts you give yourself are totally up to you, and I say, make them count! So whether it's treating yourself to different gifts every five pounds, or treating yourself to the same gift over and over (like a massage at your favorite spa), I say reward yourself over and over along the way. This mini-rewards process is a very smart way to incentivize yourself to keep going.

Finally, let's wrap things up with meal planning. The principles here are the same as with exercise. You need to plan things in advance and have a meal schedule that outlines what you're going to eat and when you're going to eat it. I'm a big fan of cooking food in advance, and many people find it easiest to set aside one night a week, usually on the weekend, to cook all the meals for the entire upcoming week. This way, you can have everything ready in the fridge to just grab and go. You should also have a reserve of healthy, high-protein snacks in places like your car and office desk. You want to go high-protein because protein is an excellent macronutrient for controlling blood sugar and staving off hunger. Foods like protein shakes, protein bars, Greek yogurt, cottage cheese, nuts and canned tuna are all high in protein and great in a pinch since they don't require much, if any, preparation. Ultimately, meal planning is all about putting yourself in the best position to avoid temptation, so when hunger does rear its head, you'll be more likely to grab your healthy meal instead of whatever junk is nearby.

MISTAKE 2
EAT MANY SMALL MEALS A DAY TO BOOST METABOLISM

YOU SAY: Eat many small meals a day to boost metabolism.

I SAY: Like many fitness myths, this idea is indeed based on some degree of fact. The thought behind the "many small meals" approach is this: Since metabolism spikes briefly in response to a meal, eating frequent small meals should keep metabolism elevated all day. Proponents of the frequent small meal approach also like to tack on that frequent meals have the added benefit of keeping you from feeling hungry, which removes the temptation to overeat.

For years, the "many small meals" regimen was preached by well-respected fitness experts and reputable magazines. At one point, I even bought into it, doing all I could to make sure I was eating or snacking every few hours during the day to keep my metabolism up. And though it was often an inconvenience to make sure I constantly had food on hand, I kept eating this way until I came across a bit of research that basically torpedoed the "many small meals" battleship.

Meal Frequency, Meal Size, and Metabolism

The digestion of food has a thermic effect, meaning that your body actually has to burn calories to break down the food you've just eaten. This thermic effect is what causes an increase in metabolism, and different types of food have different thermic effects, depending on their fat, protein, carbohydrate and fiber content. Furthermore, the exact magnitude and duration of the metabolic boost you'll experience after eating a meal is directly proportional to the size of the meal. Thus, small meals produce a small, short metabolism spike, while larger meals result in a more noticeable and longer-lasting increase in metabolism.

So the question now stands: Do many small meals, and consequently, many small metabolic spikes, result in more calories burned over a 24-hour period?

In an effort to answer this question, researchers at the French National Institute of Health and Medical Research reviewed several studies comparing metabolism to eating habits. The types of diets in these studies varied from eating just one to as many as 17 meals in a day. When all the data was collected and analyzed, the surprising result of the study was that there was no difference between the thermic effect of many small meals a day versus a few larger meals a day. Moreover, it was shown that though the two different approaches to meal frequency (many small meals versus a few larger meals) did indeed produce different metabolic boosts, by the end of each day, both meal frequency approaches balanced out in terms of overall metabolic boost and total calories burned.

Similar results were found in a study conducted at the University of Ontario where volunteers were split into two groups. One group stuck to the classic three meals per day, while the other group had three meals plus three snacks. To control for more meals in the second group, both groups were placed on a restricted calorie intake designed to stimulate weight loss. This particular study lasted eight weeks, and after reviewing the amount of fat and muscle lost during the study, researchers found no significant difference between the two groups.

Meal Frequency and Appetite Control

Now let's address the claim that several small meals can help to better control appetite. Here the science is a bit muddled and doesn't conclusively give an answer either way.

For example, one study from the University of Kansas compared six small meals against three large, protein-rich meals. More specifically, researchers sought to measure the perceived fullness of each subject after their meal. Ultimately, it was found that the three large meals left subjects feeling more satisfied by the end of the day. In another study conducted by the University of Missouri, researchers compared three meals to six meals and found similar results.

On the other hand, there are also studies that contradict these findings. In these studies, it was found that six meals per day helped dieters to feel more satisfied, which ultimately made it easier for them to stick to their diets.

So, based on the research, there doesn't seem to be one clear-cut winner with regard to appetite control.

Finding Your Balance

It seems, after looking at the research, that the decision to eat many small meals or a few big ones boils down to personal preference. That said, people often ask me how many meals I'd recommend per day, and my preference is that people eat three to four meals per day.

Why?

Because, in both my professional and personal experience, the amount of satisfaction you get from a meal has more to do with *what* you're eating, and not necessarily *when* you're eating. As far as *what,* I'm a strong advocate of low-carb diets, and I've found that when people take the time to follow a low-carb protocol, which emphasizes high intake of protein and healthy fats, these same people consistently report feeling fuller for longer periods of time than when they consume meals containing an abundance of processed and simple carbs.

Another reason I advocate a protocol of three to four meals a day is that it's a lot less complicated. Speaking from personal experience, it can become a major pain in the butt trying to schedule six healthy meals every single day. Heck, for many folks, just planning and scheduling three healthy meals a day is challenge enough. So for this reason too, I've found that many people find it easiest to stick to about three or four meals per day. Ultimately, the three-to-four meal protocol allows you to get all the fuel you need for the day without feeling stressed about constant meal planning.

Now despite my recommendation of three to four meals a day, I must stress that the best dietary protocol is the one you'll stick to for years to come. The most important thing is to find a routine that fits well with your lifestyle, instead of one that disrupts or complicates it. So if you find that eating many small meals works the best for your lifestyle, fuels your body best, and adequately controls your appetite, go that route. Either way, whatever option you choose—many small meals or a few larger meals—your ability to stick with your diet is what really matters in the long run.

MISTAKE 3

WORK YOUR ABS MORE TO GET RID OF BELLY FAT

YOU SAY: Work your abs more to get rid of belly fat.

I SAY: Attaining a sexy six-pack has become a sort of benchmark for fitness, with nearly everyone holding it up as his or her ultimate goal. And even if you could care less about having ripped abs, let's be honest, you probably wouldn't be too bothered if your stomach was flat, well-defined and chiseled.

Ever conscious of the general public's love of six-pack abs, fitness magazines make it their business to constantly advertise new abdominal workouts and nutritional supplements like fat-burning pills with "secret" ingredients that promise to help shred your belly fat. Trainers and fitness experts even specialize in ab training, flooding the internet with ebooks that tout their cutting-edge methods for helping you achieve a glorious six-pack. So yeah, without a doubt, the world is ab-obsessed.

And it makes complete sense, on the surface, that if you want a trim mid-section, you should work your abs like a beast. Unfortunately, that logic just doesn't hold up under scientific scrutiny.

Why not?

First, you need to think about the relationship of fat and muscle. Your muscles, from the day you're born, have the general anatomy that they will always have for the rest of your life. Through training, you can most certainly increase their size and strength, but the general anatomy will remain the same. And speaking of anatomy, frustratingly, your body keeps its muscles under fat. This means that no matter how big or strong your muscles are, if you have too much fat, they won't be visible. Truth be told, a six-pack is not some "mystical" thing. A six-pack is nothing more than visible muscle.

Take this fact one step further and a frightening realization emerges: Building your abs without burning fat can make your stomach actually *appear* bigger or fatter—which is terrifyingly counterproductive if you already have a pudgy belly.

Sorry ladies, Sir Mix-a-Lot was definitely wrong on this one. Skip the side bends and sit ups, because you're wasting your time.

Still don't believe me? Can't bear the thought of giving up your QVC Ab-Buster machine or your beloved crunches? Well, a study published in *The Journal of Strength and Conditioning Research* might be able to change your mind. Over the course of the six-week study, 24 healthy subjects were split into two groups. The control group did absolutely nothing to their abs, while the other group did a total of 140 reps, five days per week of various abdominal exercises.

After such an intensely focused training period, you'd expect the ab training group to have sexy, slim stomachs, right?

Nope.

There was absolutely no change in the ab workout group's overall weight, body fat percentage, or abdominal circumference. The ab group did see an increase in their ab and core muscle strength, but those precious muscles, despite their increase in strength, were still pretty much invisible because they were still hiding under pesky body fat. So what this study (and real life) teaches us is that if your body fat is too high, hours of abdominal training will prove useless if you're looking for a six-pack.

Let's make something else clear: I'm not at all saying that ab exercises are useless in general. In fact, I highly recommend exercises that engage and strengthen core and ab muscles. Why? Because as a sports doc and trainer, I'm not just about physique; I'm also about performance. And though abs have come to be viewed overall as simply "vanity muscles," there are very good reasons that it's important to actually spend time working out your abs. One major reason is that strong abdominal muscles and a strong core aid in supporting good posture and balance, while helping you through most other exercises.

That understood, you can skip the ab exercises when it comes to attaining a six-pack. But don't skip ab exercises altogether. Because as nice as it is to have a glorious six-pack, it's going to be really hard to show them off when your back is hunched and your posture's all screwed up.

Now back to six-pack abs. So how do you get those abs to show?

Simple: Take away their hiding place. This means losing body fat. Speaking in more specific terms, men should drop their body fat percentage to about 10 percent and women should shoot for about 18 percent. As unbelievably simple as that may sound, that's the big secret to getting rid of belly fat and attaining a nicely defined stomach.

As far as losing that extra body fat, yes, it sounds simple, but as any dieter knows, it's often easier said than done. Even with proper diet and exercise, belly fat is often the last bit of fat to go. Here a few extra tricks to speed up the process and help jump-start your body's fat-burning engine.

Low-Carb Dieting

Any food that you eat first needs to be stripped down to its primary building blocks before your body can absorb its nutrients. For example, protein must be broken down to amino acids. Fat will be broken down into fatty acids. And carbohydrates are broken down into glucose. Glucose is just one source of fuel that our bodies use to power things like brain function and muscle contractions.

During the day, people eat a variety of foods containing mixtures of protein, fats and carbs. But for the purposes of this discussion, I want you to ignore fats and protein and just focus your attention on carbs. Carbs are a very important macronutrient to hone in on when it comes to accelerating fat loss. As I mentioned earlier, when you eat food containing carbohydrates, your body will break down the carbs to glucose. Then, to make sure that this glucose gets to where it needs to go and doesn't just float around in your blood stream, your pancreas will release insulin, an important hormone that helps shuttle glucose into your body's liver, muscle cells, fat cells and other tissues that want to use all that glucose for fuel.

In your liver and muscles, glucose is used for immediate energy. However, if more glucose is provided than is actually needed, your liver and muscle cells will convert the excess glucose to glycogen, which is a storage form of glucose that can be used at a later time.

However, things are a little different when glucose enters your fat cells. When glucose enters our fat cells, they will begin working to turn that glucose into triglycerides and *more* fat—not glycogen. *You may also recognize triglycerides as something constantly mentioned when doctors talk about things like obesity, heart disease and other not-so-pleasant medical conditions.* So eating carbohydrates—or more specifically, certain types of carbohydrates—in abundance, can have long-term negative effects such as high triglyceride levels, in addition to contributing to the expansion of your waistline.

Getting back to insulin—*I want you to really pay attention here* because insulin is a very important hormone that you absolutely need to understand in terms of weight loss, or more specifically, fat loss. Insulin is so important because it has an inverse relationship to your body's ability to burn fat. In other words, when insulin is high, fat burn stops. Furthermore, insulin will actually stimulate your body to store fat. On the other hand, when insulin drops low below a certain threshold, fat burn kicks in. This phenomenon is the whole basis for low-carb diets. The whole rationale for low-carb, and it's a pretty brilliant one too, is still to eat, but to primarily consume foods that don't elevate blood sugar and insulin levels so that the body is regularly in a state of wanting to burn fat. The low-carb dieter is very careful about the amount and type of carbs she eats, while eating a diet that is plentiful in healthy fats and protein because these two macronutrients don't have a significant effect on insulin like carbs do.

The result of eating low-carb is ultimately **accelerated fat loss**, so going low-carb is a fantastic way to help shred belly fat.

Important note: I'm not at all saying that low-carb is the *only* kind of diet to help you lose weight and belly fat, so if you don't want to try the low-carb route, don't. Overall, people think abs are made in the gym, but they're wrong. Abs are made in the kitchen. So whether it's low-carb, Paleo, calorie-restricted, or whatever, if you want to effectively lose body fat and get a six-pack, it's an irrefutable fact that you will need to get your diet in check.

Fasted Training

Now back to *when* we eat. When you eat a meal, your body goes into a state where it will be working to break down the nutrients from your food so it can put those nutrients to good use. When you eat, insulin becomes elevated, suppressing your body's ability to burn fat. One more thing: It's important to remember that insulin is always going to be released to some degree, great or small, after you eat a meal, most especially one that is carb-dense. But as I mentioned earlier, insulin and fat burn have this inverse, antagonistic relationship. So if you choose not to eat anything at all, insulin levels are going to remain low. In this state, called "fasting," insulin isn't around to exert its suppressive effect, and your body will once again flip its switch and start burning some of its fat stores.

Once your body is in a fasted state, you're now in the perfect window for a fat-torching workout. Fat burn during the fasted state is especially amplified with weightlifting or strength training, which not only gets your body burning excess calories but also keeps it in that increased fat-burning mode for as much as 24 hours after you've finished your workout. This ongoing fat burn is also known as the "afterburn effect," and strength training is something I seriously advise people to get involved in if they're serious about dropping body fat.

Something else to keep in mind is that the benefits of fasted training are enhanced even more if you've abstained from food for at least six hours. Since it may be difficult to fast for six solid hours during the day, one simple solution is to exercise first thing in the morning before you've broken your fast.

Fun Fact: The word "breakfast" comes from the phrase "to break a fast."

Now I realize that all this talk of fasted training may send up some red flags, especially if you've listened to advice along the lines of "you should eat something before you exercise so you don't get dizzy from low blood sugar," or "you should eat something before you exercise so you'll have energy to get through your workout." Regardless of what you may or may not have heard, I can assure you that fasted training is perfectly safe. In fact, it's one of the smartest and most efficient ways to speed up fat loss. So assuming you don't have medical issues where your doctor has specifically advise against it, there's nothing wrong with exercising on an empty stomach.

Green Tea Extract

While the market is definitely flooded with useless fat-burning supplements, you will be thrilled to learn that not all fat-burning supplements out there are complete snake oil. Green tea extract is one of the pretty good ones, hence the widespread popularity of green tea fat-burning supplements.

Green tea extract is an herbal product derived from green tea leaves, and green tea extract is a commonly sought-after fat burner because it contains a large amount of powerful antioxidants called catechins. Catechins provide a ton of health benefits, one of which is accelerated fat loss—particularly fat loss around the abdominal area. You should know though, that these fat-burning benefits of catechins have only been shown to be significant when combined with exercise. It's also important to note that based on research, an effective dose of catechins hovers somewhere between 600 to 900 mg per day. The average green tea extract will contain about 300 mg of catechins per pill, so this would mean having to take two to three green tea extract pills per day to reap the fat-burning effects of catechins. Mind you, I'm talking averages here. Reality is there are literally hundreds of green tea extract products on the market and the potency of catechins will vary from product to product. So the amount of green tea extract pills you'll have to take to get those 600 to 900 mg of catechins will vary and will be greatly determined by the quality of the green tea supplement you purchase.

*Visit my online store at **DrPhoenyx.com** to learn more about my energy and performance supplement, *BodyElite*. *BodyElite* is one of my premium nutritional supplements, specially formulated to improve exercise performance, boost metabolism and assist with healthy weight loss.

MISTAKE 4

LOW-CARB DIETS ARE TOO HARD TO STICK TO

YOU SAY: Low-carb diets are too hard to stick to.

I SAY: Low-carb diets still aren't a common recommendation by dieticians or mainstream fitness professionals, even despite the success of low-carb plans like Atkins, which spurred the low-carb craze. Although it isn't one of the most "conventional" diets, it may surprise you to know that people have been eating low-carb with ease for thousands of years, and thankfully low-carb doesn't show any signs of going extinct. And make no mistake, the longevity and popularity of the low-carb diet continues for one very simple reason: Because it works—really, really well in fact!

Even though it has proven quite effective at helping people slim down, the low-carb lifestyle still has its naysayers. Interestingly enough, the naysayers rarely claim that low-carb diets "don't work." That argument definitely wouldn't hold water because the effectiveness of low-carb has been solidly established by research. Instead, critics make another assertion to bash low-carb. They say that low-carb diets are just too hard to stick to for any length of time to have any real, lasting effect on your waistline. To further bolster their claims, critics often spew rhetoric like, "Low-carb isn't healthy because you have to eliminate *all* carbs from your diet, and carbs are an essential food group."

At first glance, this argument may hold some weight and be enough to frighten off most dieters. The thought of giving up an entire "essential" food group that also contains delicious foods like baked goods, sweets, and fried goodies can be too much for some to handle. Carbs stir and soothe our emotions, and it's no coincidence that a ton of carb-ilicious foods are thought of as "comfort foods." For some people, the mere thought of cutting back on carbs is like a dietary death sentence. But for savvy dieters, or at least the ones with an understanding of basic nutrition, it'll be quite obvious that the whole "low-carb is unhealthy" or "low-carb is too difficult" arguments are just frivolous scare tactics and diet propaganda.

Nutrition 101: Macronutrients and the Truth about Carbs

All food is made up of one or a combination of three primary macronutrients—protein, fat, and carbohydrates. Unbeknownst to many people, only two of these macronutrients are essential to sustaining human life. Can you guess which one isn't?

If you guessed protein or fat, you'd be wrong. Carbohydrates are the only macronutrient that is not necessary to sustain life. Yes, as many of you know, carbohydrates do provide glucose and energy that the body uses, but the body can also derive its energy just from fats and protein. Furthermore, when deprived of carbs, the body can actually take fats and protein and convert them into glucose via a process called *gluconeogenesis*. It's really incredible that our bodies can do this, and gluconeogenesis is a perfectly normal and healthy process. So contrary to what you've been told, carbohydrates are not an essential food group.

Moreover, the low-carb diet protocol actually doesn't seek to eliminate *all* carbs. For those who don't know, foods like spinach, kale and broccoli do contain carbs, and the low-carb protocol actually advocates that you stuff yourself with these types of food. What low-carb specifically seeks to eliminate (or drastically reduce) is what are known as *processed* carbs and sugar. Processed carbs are far from essential, and moreover, processed carbs and sugar are the main culprits behind many of the health issues we see today like obesity, diabetes and heart disease. When I say processed carbs, I'm talking about all those breads, breakfast cereals, grains, pastries, pastas, and other carb-ilicious goodies. This is what you'll be giving up, or better said, this is what you'll be severely restricting on low-carb. Because the truth is, on low-carb you certainly are allowed to treat yourself to these types of foods occasionally, just not every day like many of you are currently used to.

As far as what you *can* eat regularly on low-carb, that's far from "restricted." On low-carb you'll be eating tons of lean and fatty meats, from chicken to pork. You'll be eating lots of healthy fats from things like butter, olive oil and coconut oil. You will also be eating heaps of low-carb veggies like broccoli, cauliflower, spinach, kale, Brussels sprouts, cabbage, Swiss chard, lettuce, cucumber, celery, mushrooms, avocado, squash, zucchini, pumpkin, and on and on and on. Now, do all these food options sound like you'll be starving?

Nope!

Why Traditional Diets Fall Short

When you think of "traditional" dieting, this is probably the protocol that comes to mind:

1. Removing as much fat as you can from your diet, and

2. Drastically restricting daily calorie intake, which commonly leads to perpetual hunger and sheer misery

Several randomized controlled studies have pitted low-carb diets against the type of "traditional" diet protocol above, and you know what the results were? Can you guess which diet was the better option in terms of ease and long-term weight loss? If you guessed low-carb you'd be right.

But how can this be?

How could low-carb actually be *easier* to follow?

You've been told by everyone else that low-carb is really hard to follow.

You've been told low-carb cuts out an entire, essential food group.

What's the real deal?

The real deal is, any diet that can only be followed for a short period of time and does nothing to elicit any real, lasting lifestyle change in the dieter will ultimately be ineffective. That's why all those fad diets you come across, which are purposefully designed for rapid, short-term weight loss, are essentially a wash and just a complete waste of your time. Sure, you'll lose some weight by eating nothing but grapefruit. But trust and believe, you'll gain all that weight back as soon as you reenter the real world and old eating habits resurface. This is where low-carb is drastically different. Low-carb is not a fad. It is not a "short term" solution. Low-carb is a diet that can be comfortably followed for life. And despite calling it a diet, I like to think of low-carb as a lifestyle because the word "diet" in itself tends to carry the connotation of being a "temporary" solution.

Last, but definitely not least, low-carb cuts through the BS, propaganda, and all the flat-out lies and misinformation you've been told about nutrition and dieting.

When you decide to learn about and go low-carb, you'll finally have the master key to weight loss and overall health.

But don't take my word for it. Listen to the science.

Less Hunger Means Less Eating

Low-carb diets take advantage of several physiological mechanisms to help you lose weight, the most famous of these being "ketosis." In the most basic of terms, ketosis is a fabulous physiological state where the human body literally runs on its fat stores, *24-7*. Pause for a moment to take that in.

Through low-carb dieting and ketosis, your body will literally burn off body fat *irrespective* of exercise. *Sounds pretty sweet, huh?*

Like I mentioned earlier, carbs are not essential for human function, and if you restrict carbs long enough, your body will eventually enter a state where it's forced to start using your fat stores as fuel.

And it doesn't end there!

There's another, lesser-known "side effect" that comes with eating a low-carb diet—a side effect that will actually make it *easier* for you to stick with it: You'll be less hungry.

Why will you be less hungry? Well, for several reasons. Here are three major ones:

1. Your diet will consist of more protein and fats, which have a more satiating effect than carbs.

2. Low-carb diets better regulate insulin and blood sugar levels, thus more effectively controlling hunger.

3. By eating low-carb and entering ketosis, your body will start converting fat to something called "ketone bodies," which have an appetite suppressing effect.

According to a study published in *The Journal of Clinical Endocrinology and Metabolism*, low-carbers lost more weight even though they ate until they were completely full. In fact, the low-carb dieters often weren't able to eat as much as they wanted because they got full rather quickly. These are just a handful of the many benefits that give low-carb diets a major advantage over "traditional diets," which normally leave people feeling hungry and unsatisfied. And let's be honest, it's the traditional "low-calorie, low-fat diet" that regularly leaves people feeling hungry and unsatisfied, and thus more likely to fall off the wagon.

So imagine that. A diet that doesn't require you to drastically cut calories, that suppresses hunger, that gives you the ability to actually eat until satisfied, and that promises more significant weight loss.

This isn't a dream, people. This is low-carb.

Jump Right In

Truth is, I can throw studies and facts and data at you all day, but you won't fully trust what I'm saying until you try it out for yourself. So if you've been skeptical or just plain curious about low-carb, I say give it a try for just 30 days. *Sixty days if you really want to be bad-ass!*

Try it out and see how you feel and look after 30 or 60 days. By that point, your body will have adjusted to lower processed carbs and sugar intake, you will have adopted a meal plan of your favorite low-carb foods, and you'll start to see all the positive effects on your body. The positive effects of low-carb really are astounding, and hand to God, it's not uncommon for folks to drop 10-plus pounds in their first month of going low-carb. Plus, you'll notice that once processed carbs like grains and sweets are taken out of the bulk of your diet, your taste buds will change and your cravings for these types of foods will subside. For example, it's not uncommon to discover after going low-carb that foods like carrots, which might have tasted like chalk before, will now be much sweeter when you bite into them. Plus, low-carb will enable you to explore many other food options and recipes that you'll surely end up loving.

So as scary and skeptical as it might sound, low-carb isn't the devil like you've been told. But the best way to realize this for yourself and get all the benefits of the low-carb diet is just to jump in and give it a try.

MISTAKE 5
FOR FASTER FAT LOSS, EXERCISE AS OFTEN AS POSSIBLE, FOR AS LONG AS POSSIBLE

YOU SAY: For faster fat loss, exercise as often as possible, for as long as possible.

I SAY: People often believe that the more they exercise, and the longer their workouts are, the faster they'll lose weight. And I can see how this would make sense. This is, after all, the way just about everything else in your life works.

If you want to make more money or advance further in your career, you work more. If you want to get better grades, you study more. If you want to become the next Jimi Hendrix, you practice your guitar more. Overall, it's a completely logical rule of thumb that success comes with consistent, hard work.

Unfortunately, our bodies don't totally work that way. When it comes to fitness, or more specifically, weight loss, too much, too often can start to become counterproductive. Yes, you read that right. Too much exercise can actually backfire. There does come a point when all those non-stop hours spent in the gym become useless, or worse yet, detrimental to your physique. This is especially true with weightlifting and cardio.

Why is this so? How can someone spend so much time in the gym and end up not having much to show for it?

Because fat loss, muscle growth, and overall body transformation aren't just a result of work or exercise. They are also the result of rest and recovery. Your body is stimulated to burn fat when key hormones are in balance, and your muscles grow not *during* the actual training session, but *afterwards* when you allow them to properly rest to recover. So ultimately, overtraining compromises fat loss and muscle growth because it throws off your hormones and the time your body needs to rebuild itself.

Slowed Fat Loss

You don't need me to tell you that it would absolutely suck if you spent hours upon hours working out and all you had to show for it were clothes that still fit too tight and a pudgy belly. I mean, that's precisely the opposite of what we're going for, right?

Well, when you overtrain, this is precisely what will happen. Overtraining will affect your body's hormone levels, resulting in slowed fat loss. There are two key hormones that end up being thrown out of whack with overtraining—testosterone and cortisol. In the case of testosterone, if overtraining persists, this hormone's levels will dip, and over time, gradual muscle loss will occur. Muscle loss is one of the worst things that can happen to an individual trying to lose weight. Muscle is key for boosting metabolic rate, calorie burn, and ultimately, fat metabolism. Muscle is indeed your greatest fat burner, and testosterone is a key hormone for stimulating muscle growth.

In the case of cortisol, overtraining has been shown to increase plasma cortisol levels by up to 43 percent. Among other effects, cortisol suppresses the immune system, decreases bone formation, and can lead to weight gain.

Not-so-Fun Fact: Generally called "the stress hormone," cortisol is famously known for stimulating the storage of belly fat, so overtraining can result in difficulty losing belly fat. Even worse, cortisol has a catabolic effective, meaning that it destroys muscle too—a double whammy for fat loss.

Signs of Overtraining

So how common is overtraining really? And how do you know if you're overtraining?

The fact is, many people at the gym have periods of time where they're likely to overtrain. If you're someone who just loves to exercise and feels compelled to exercise often, you may end up overtraining because you're constantly chasing that fantastic post-workout high. Those endorphins from breaking a good sweat can become absolutely addictive, and I'm definitely guilty of "chasing the high." Also, if you're someone who has a lot of weight to lose, especially in a short period of time, the temptation to overtrain can become hard to resist. Think about that woman who's at the gym every day for hours at a time, rotating between treadmill, stationary bike and elliptical. Yet interestingly enough, you notice that her physique never really improves, even after months of exercise. She's doing all this work, but not making any progress. That is a classic case of overtraining, and maybe that woman is you.

To avoid overtraining, I tell people that regardless of your fitness level or fitness goals, it's wise to cap your workout sessions at no longer than two hours at a time. After two hours of consistent exercise, cortisol levels will start to rise and the risk of overtraining will greatly increase. Last but not least, to both treat and prevent overtraining, it's very important that you get a good night's sleep every night so that your body has time to recover and that you eat properly so that your muscles have everything they need to repair themselves.

Also you should look out for these signs of overtraining: chronic fatigue, chronic pain, underperformance and even depression. Overtrained individuals will feel weaker, less energetic and less focused during their workout. To their great frustration, they won't be able to perform the way they normally would. Maybe they can't lift as much or run as fast as they could on previous days. Or they may notice aches and pains that take a lot longer to subside or don't subside at all. They may no longer get that invigorating post-workout high and instead feel tired, moody and uncomfortable after their workouts.

These are just some of the signs of overtraining. If you spot just one of these symptoms on its own, that won't necessarily mean that you're overtraining, so don't panic. However, if you're experiencing several of these symptoms all at once, chances are pretty good that you should take a couple days (or longer) off from your workout schedule. As heartbreaking as that might be, it'll be necessary to get you back to 100 percent. At the end of the day, exercise should lift your mood and energize your body, so if it does the opposite, you need to take some time off.

How to Properly Rest and Recover

Ultimately, the number of rest days you need during the week will depend on you, your training style and your fitness level. Some people train very intensely and may need two days off per week, while for others, one day may be enough. As a general rule of thumb, I advise giving yourself at least one day off a week. However, if you've noticed that you're suffering from two or more signs of overtraining that I mentioned earlier, I'd advise taking a week completely off to let your body fully rest and recover. If your issues persist after a week of rest, consider seeing a doctor. And once you do decide to get back to training, I'd strongly advise making some changes to your workout routine to avoid the same problems again.

Now I want to share a bit of information that I'm sure some of you will be very, very happy to receive, especially all you workout warriors who can't stand the idea of taking even one day off a week from exercise. For folks (like myself) who don't really like the idea of spending a whole day being inactive, there is a form of rest and recovery that actually allows you to exercise. It's called "active recovery." Put simply, active recovery, or "active rest," is sort of a hybrid between passive recovery (i.e. rest) and exercise. Active recovery involves exercising on purpose as a means of helping your body recover, and the guidelines of active recovery are simple. You can do pretty much any type of exercise, as long as you keep your exercise intensity low.

Examples of active recovery include things like walking and yoga. Active recovery is something I regularly practice and it's something I highly recommend to people who enjoy being very active. Interestingly enough, a growing body of research shows that active recovery may even be *better* than passive recovery in terms of resolving muscle soreness, expediting muscle recovery and repair, and enhancing psychological and mental recovery, as well as promoting mental and physical relaxation.

MISTAKE 6
EATING FAT WILL MAKE YOU FAT

YOU SAY: Eating fat will make you fat.

I SAY: Here's the bottom line: Eating fat will not make you fat or sick.

As is often the case with fitness myths, the belief that "eating fat will make you fat" came into being from a bit of truth based on hard science. Problem was, that truth was grossly misinterpreted.

So why do so many people believe that fat is bad, will make you fat or sick and cause things like heart attacks? Basically, this all started decades ago, particularly due to a research study known as the Seven Countries Study, which helped spur the "fat will make you fat" myth. This bit of research, which examined heart risk based on lifestyle and dietary habits, found that there were more cases of heart disease in countries where people ate more fat, especially saturated fat. Thus it was concluded that fat caused heart disease. But here's the problem with this study: Correlation is not causation. And just because both fat intake and heart disease were higher among the same population doesn't mean the heart disease was caused by the fat consumption. Here's another way to look at it: Every day you wake up and the sun comes up, right? But just because these two events happen at the same time doesn't mean one causes the other. In other words, you waking up doesn't cause the sun to come up. By that same token, it was also wrong for health experts to conclude based on the Seven Countries Study that fat consumption caused heart disease.

Because of similar research to the Seven Countries Study, health professionals continued to make faulty associations between fat consumption and conditions like obesity and heart disease. Fortunately, that's all changed with more research and better research analysis. And now it's become quite clear that the true culprit behind conditions like obesity is actually sugar, not fat. Moreover, a review of all the research on saturated fat published in *The American Journal of Clinical Nutrition* found there was no correlation between saturated fat and heart disease.

The Skinny on Getting Fat

The mechanism of weight gain and weight loss is about the interaction of both calories *and* hormones—or more specifically calories and insulin. Fact is, the only way to lose weight is to burn off more calories than you eat, or to create what is known as a "caloric deficit." Likewise, to gain weight, you will need to create a "caloric surplus" by eating more calories than you burn off. Furthermore, the mechanism of fat storage is caused by the hormone insulin, not dietary fat itself. In fact, if you were to actually look at and compare the subsequent insulin responses of each macronutrient, you'd find that the consumption of fat (and protein) does not trigger the hormonal response that creates fat storage the way the consumption of sugar and processed carbohydrates does.

So while it may be a bit reflexive to *think* that eating fat will make you fat—just by sheer virtue of the name "fat"—science has shown that this just isn't the case. Eating fat, especially saturated fat, has indeed gotten a bad rap for a long time. Fortunately, health professionals have learned the error of our ways, and we're now turning our attention to the real enemies: sugar and processed carbs.

So if you've had difficulty losing weight, or if you just want to be healthier overall, I'd strongly advise that you look into revamping your diet so that it consists primarily of protein, healthy fats, and minimal sugar.

Here are a few of my favorite sources of healthy fat:

- Avocados – Pass the guacamole, *por favor!*

- Nuts – Brazil nuts, almonds, walnuts, pecans and macadamia nuts

- Seeds – sunflower, pumpkin, sesame, chia, flax and hemp

- Fatty fish that are rich in omega-3 fats – wild salmon, sardines, mackerel, and herring

- Grass-fed or sustainably raised animal products like grass-fed beef and free-range chicken (Check out the Environmental Working Group's Meat Eater's Guide for a list of animal products that are good for you and good for the planet.)

- Extra virgin coconut oil, which is a great plant-based source of saturated fat and one of the healthiest fats you can eat and cook with. Numerous studies have found extra virgin coconut oil to have the following benefits:

    Improves heart health

    Boosts thyroid function

    Supports immune function

    Increases metabolism

    Promotes weight loss

Before closing, I wanted to mention another benefit of eating a diet high in healthy fat: satiation. Because the digestion of fats strongly stimulates satiation, people on high-fat diets find that they tend to experience less hunger even with reduced caloric intake. Interestingly enough, this does not seem to be the case with low-fat diets, and the fat-satiation correlation is one of the main reasons why low-fat diets are doomed to fail and require such a higher exercise of fierce willpower. In fact, it's not uncommon for people on low-fat diets to feel constantly hungry because their hunger never seems satisfied without fat, even when they still consume more calories. So, another benefit to eating fat is that it makes you fuller sooner and longer.

Bottom line: Eating fat doesn't make you fat. Eating sugar is what makes you fat. Furthermore, eating a diet that's rich in healthy fats can actually help you feel more satisfied, which in turn helps you lose weight and keep it off.

MISTAKE 7
WOMEN WILL GET BULKY FROM LIFTING HEAVY WEIGHTS

YOU SAY: Women will get bulky from lifting heavy weights.

I SAY: Generally speaking, most women want the same type of body. They don't want to be too bulky or too thin. They want lean, toned, defined muscles, especially in their legs and arms. They want a slim waist and a flat tummy, with sexy, subtle muscle definition in their abs. And most important of all, they want a tight, round, onion booty.

Onion booty (noun): a booty so fine it'll make you want to cry.

Essentially, the body type that most women want is, *in fact,* an athletic build. And the fact is, this athletic build—onion booty and all—isn't just the result of losing body fat. It's the result of losing body fat *and* building just enough muscle in all the right places.

For example, when most women want to lose weight, they focus heavily on jogging for hours on the treadmill or incessantly working out on the elliptical (basically, nothing but steady-state cardio), while totally ignoring any type of muscle-building exercises like squats, lunges, or plain ol' weightlifting.

Ultimately, the result of this exercise protocol will be a body that just looks plain skinny, or even worse, a body that looks "skinny-fat." Skinny-fat is a term used to describe a skinny individual whose body has a flabby, undefined look because, due to lack of strength training, there's very little muscle tone or definition. If you've ever seen a "skinny-fat" person, you know how unappealing this type of physique can be. Think *pancake booty* instead of *onion booty*. Believe you me, skinny-fat is not a good look. So for ladies who want a slim *and* sexy physique, you will need to focus not just on dropping body fat, but also on building muscle to give your body curves in the all right places.

When I ask women who are trying to lose weight why they spend more time on things like the treadmill and almost no time at all lifting weight, the answer is the same 99.9 percent of the time: *Because I don't want to get bulky.*

Even the ladies who do actually lift weights attempt to follow a training style to avoid getting the dreaded "bulky" look. Often their "anti-bulky" training style comprises lifting very light weights for many reps. They do this because they've been taught to believe that light weights are all you need for "toned" muscles. They look at the big, "swole" dudes in the gym lifting heavy weights and they figure, "I want to tone up, but not *that* much," and they ultimately reason that the solution is to lift, but lift lighter. Unfortunately, this entire strategy and line of reasoning is completely wrong.

So let's clear up all this confusion by forever squashing the whole fear of bulking up. First of all, bulking up is extremely difficult to do— for women *as well as* for men—but most especially for women, the reasoning being that women, due to our hormones, are at a distinct biological disadvantage when it comes to building muscle like men. The hormone primarily responsible for muscle production is testosterone, and the average woman produces a mere five to 10 percent of the testosterone of the average man. In fact, one study found that post-exercise testosterone levels in men were an incredible 45 percent higher than in women. Some research even suggests that women's bodies don't produce any extra testosterone at all after exercise, but instead respond by cranking out human growth hormone, estradiol and cortisol.

All this talk of hormones simply means that women are built to respond to exercise in a very different way than men. More specifically, women's bodies function in such a way that heavy lifting doesn't necessarily increase the size of muscles as much as it improves muscle strength and endurance.

Now, for you ladies pointing to female bodybuilders and questioning how or why their bodies can end up looking so muscular, you need to recognize that female bodybuilders are not representative of the average dieter or the average gym rat. Female bodybuilders follow an insanely regimented fitness protocol, and it can literally take up to a year of a rigidly designed workout routine, coupled with a very strict diet, to build the amount of muscle that female bodybuilders have, and that the average woman may fear. Ladies, trust me on this: You will never wake up one day after a few weeks of lifting heavy weights and be completely taken by surprise by your bulging biceps, linebacker shoulders or rippling leg muscles. That's just not how it works.

Fun Fact: Muscle has only 35 percent the mass of fat. So the reality is, if you were to build two pounds of muscle and lose two pounds of body fat, you would actually be smaller than you were before even though you weigh the same.

Another point against the "anti-bulky" protocol of low weights for high reps is rooted in a physiological effect known as muscle adaptation. Muscle adaptation is something that occurs naturally after lifting a certain weight over time. For example, after a few days or a few weeks, your muscles will end up adapting to whatever challenge you're putting them up against. While those 20-pound dumbbells may be difficult to lift now, over time, you will notice that the weights become pretty easy to lift. What has happened is that your muscles have adapted to the weight. And although you might continue to burn some extra calories by doing tons of reps with this easy 20-pound weight, you ultimately won't see much change in the muscle tone of your arms because you are no longer challenging your muscles. For this reason, you'll need to progressively increase weight as you train, as well as lift heavier in general. Remember, it's the challenge that spurs the change and builds the muscle tone and shape you're looking for.

More Selling Points

Alright, so it's now been pretty much established that building muscle can satisfy all of your vanity and get you that hot physique you've always wanted. But there are also much more health-conscious reasons to lift heavy than just looking like a warrior goddess.

For one thing, you'll age better. As the years go by, it's typical for women to lose mobility and have difficulty maintaining a healthy weight. The reason for this process is loss of lean muscle mass.

You may be surprised to learn that, unless you do something to stop it, starting in your 20's, your body loses a small amount of muscle and strength every year. Research has shown that upwards of 40 percent of total muscle is lost between the ages of 20 and 60. In medical lingo, muscle loss is known as "sarcopenia," and studies have associated gradual loss of muscle with numerous health problems and weight gain.

Remember, muscle is what burns fat, so with less muscle as you age, it will be harder to keep body fat low. However, by lifting weights and keeping your muscle mass up, you'll keep your body lean while counteracting many other negative effects of aging.

One study conducted at The University of Texas highlighted a wide range of additional health benefits that women reap from lifting weights. It was found that women who lift weights have a reduced risk of developing diabetes, heart disease, and even cancer. Women who lift weights are also at a significantly lower risk for developing osteoporosis (bone loss) as they age. Last, but definitely not least, as mentioned earlier, since muscle burns calories (even when you're not moving), women who lift weights and focus on building muscle into old age will enjoy the benefit of keeping their metabolism up and their weight down.

All of the above is precisely why I strongly believe that *everyone*, both men and women of all ages, should include some form of strength training in his or her exercise routine. The frequency and intensity of the training should be dictated by your personal exercise goals, but even if the goal is just to stay healthy, strength training should be part of your regimen.

How to Do It

So we've established that you should lift heavy to improve your physique as well as your overall health. But what's "heavy"? Do you need to be lifting the same weight as the super-swole guy doing 200-pound bench presses?

Not at all! (*I hear you breathing a huge sigh of relief*)

What constitutes "heavy" can be pretty subjective. So to make things more objective, as a rule of thumb, when I say "lift heavy," what I mean is to use a weight that you can only lift eight to 10 times before your muscles become totally fatigued and you can't possibly lift that weight one more time. If, however, you find that you can do more than 10 reps with a given weight, you'll need to make it heavier.

Heavy weights really are one of the best tools for total body transformation. And when it comes to toning up, my personal mantra is, "*Get mean to get lean!*"

So ladies, it's time to drop those cutesy, padded pink dumbbells, grab some of those heavy weights, and get a lil' nasty like the boys. For toned, sexy legs, you're going to focus on those scary-looking "man lifts" like squats, deadlifts and barbell lunges. For lean, beautiful arms, add in some pull-ups, dips and heavy biceps curls with weighted bars rather than light dumbbells. These are just a handful of the many, many exercises that'll leave you looking fantastic and on a path to long-lasting health.

Bottom line: When you lift heavy, your muscles get stronger (but not necessarily bigger). Now ladies, if you pump yourself full of testosterone, eat way more calories than you are burning every day, and lift heavy weights, then you will certainly get bigger.

But if you lift heavy while eating healthy foods at a caloric deficit, your muscles will get stronger and denser. You will also burn the fat on top of your muscles, and you will get that sexy, "toned" look that you're after.

MISTAKE 8

FRUIT JUICE AND FRUIT SMOOTHIES ARE HEALTHY

YOU SAY: Fruit juice and fruit smoothies are healthy.

I SAY: In an effort to get more servings of fruit in their diet, many people turn to drinking fruit juices and fruit smoothies. Sometimes these beverages are made at home with beautiful and expensive chromed-out appliances, and sometimes these fruit drinks are bought at the local Jamba Juice or prepackaged from the local grocery store.

The most common reason that I've heard from people who are gung-ho about juicing is based on the idea that juicing leaves you with a liquid concentrate that's more nutritious than whole foods in terms of vitamin, mineral and antioxidant content. And while this might be true (actually it isn't), there are many problems that can arise when you go the route of juicing.

Downsides of Juicing

Here's a list of potential drawbacks to juicing:

You may not get enough fiber. One problem that arises with juicing is due to the mechanism of juicing itself. Juicers work to extract portions of fruit and vegetables like the skin and the pulp. Or some people may remove the peel from produce themselves before feeding into the juicer. And therein lies the problem. The skin and pulp of fruits and vegetables are where you'll find the bulk of their fiber, so by juicing, you'll miss out on the health benefits of fiber. Incidentally, fiber is in short supply in most of our diets already. Still, juicing proponents argue that removing this fiber helps the body absorb nutrients more easily, but that's simply not true. Your body needs fiber to promote healthy digestive function and fiber helps fill you up better than juice alone.

Juices aren't miracle cancer cures. This information might come as a shock, especially with all the talk about the miracles of juicing, but according to the American Cancer Society, "There is no convincing scientific evidence that extracted juices are healthier than whole foods."

Juicing can be expensive. Look, I'll never be one to compromise the quality of my foods to save a buck. I do juice myself, but that doesn't mean that I'm totally oblivious to the fact that it takes a fairly high volume of produce to make even a small volume of juice. Furthermore, if you want to get the most bang for your buck, you're going to have to invest in a high-quality juice extractor—which won't be cheap. When you add all this together, juicing can become quite expensive. And depending on how frequently you juice, and *why* you're actually doing it, the costs of juicing may begin to outweigh the benefits.

The Blood Sugar Conundrum

Still, the loss of fiber and the other downsides I mentioned above aren't even the biggest cause for concern when it comes to juices and smoothies. The real concern is sugar.

Regularly juicing high-glycemic fruits like pineapple or watermelon, especially in combination with a low-fiber diet, can set you up for frequent blood sugar spikes. Furthermore, for those of you looking to try juice fasts as a way to lose weight, this method could prove problematic, since homemade juices from some fruits and vegetables can contain more natural sugar than you might realize, thus adding a surprisingly high number of calories and thwarting efforts to drop

And That's Why You're Fat

pounds. Plus, as I mentioned earlier, the fact that juices tend to lack fiber complicates matters even further, since fiber-poor foods tend to be less filling, which sets you up for feeling hungrier and less satisfied.

Now back to sugar.

In the case of store-bought juices and smoothies, it's not uncommon for manufacturers to literally pack these types of drinks with sugar and, in worst-case scenarios, high-fructose corn syrup. This is all done in a very purposeful effort to make the drinks more palatable and keep you coming back for more.

For example, a 2012 study looked at 187 products including juices, smoothies (juice that includes the pulp), fruit drinks (water and fruit juice), and fruit-flavored waters (which contain no juice). The study subsequently found that 71 percent of all of these beverages contained added sugar. Honestly, that may not even be very surprising to most people, but what will really blow your hair back is how little juice these beverages actually contained. In the case of the smoothies, they only contained 44.5 percent fruit juice, and the so-called "fruit juices" only contained an embarrassing 10.5 percent fruit juice.

As far as sugar content, on average, the fruit-flavored waters contained 5.7 grams of sugar per 8-ounce serving, and the fruit juices and fruit smoothies both came in at a whopping 25.92 grams of sugar in every 8-ounce glass.

In my opinion, downing these types of fruit beverages is no different from literally strapping an IV to your arm and giving yourself an infusion of straight sugar. So what I'm about to share now should come as no surprise: Research has subsequently found that regularly drinking these types of fruit juice beverages has been linked to an increased risk of developing diabetes.

The Real Squeeze

When you take all this into consideration and really weigh the pros versus the cons, you'll see that there's nothing significantly healthier about fruit juice and fruit smoothies when compared to eating whole foods. In most cases, I believe you'll be much better off primarily sticking to whole fruits and vegetables. And if you do choose to juice, a better strategy is to juice mostly vegetables, adding only a small amount of fruit for sweetness. This method won't resolve the issue of lost fiber, but it will significantly control the sugar content of your juice or smoothie.

Bottom line: Freshly extracted juices from all types of produce can be part of a healthy diet in moderate amounts. Remember though, juices are not fundamentally healthier than whole fruits or vegetables. And as long as you eat a balanced diet rich with whole foods, you can rest assured that you're going to get plenty of vitamins, minerals and nutrients, as well as fiber.

MISTAKE 9
IT'S OK TO HOLD ONTO CARDIO MACHINES WHILE EXERCISING

YOU SAY: It's OK to hold onto cardio machines while exercising.

I SAY: I spend a considerable amount of my time at the gym, so obviously I see a huge number of able-bodied people, of all ages, chugging away on the cardio machines hour after hour, day after day, week after week, and, yes, year after year.

Which now leads me to one of the utter banes of my existence. To me it's like fingernails on a chalkboard, or the sound of Gilbert Gottfried whispering sweet nothings in my ear.

I'm talking about people who hold onto the StairMaster, elliptical or treadmill when exercising. Worse yet, whether these people are moving at a turtle's pace or full on sprinting, they're leaning over, holding onto the handlebars or console for dear life as if they cannot trust themselves to support their own body weight and not suddenly fly off the back of the treadmill into a deluxe face plant. I've even seen people running on the treadmill for an *entire* workout while holding onto the handlebars. I'm talking over 30 minutes of running and handlebar holding! That's just wrong on so many levels! For one, it's terrible form because your back is rounded and your spine doesn't get enough support. Second, it just makes my eyes hurt to watch.

Fact is, the compulsive need that so many gym-goers have to hold onto the cardio equipment is purely psychological. Mind you, these are the same women who are doing unsupported lunges and squats and even deadlifts. They also take group exercise classes like Zumba and boot camp, so I know that these women have the coordination it takes to swing their arms and put one foot in front of the other without assistance.

So now I'm telling you like I tell all my clients. Whether going slow or fast, you want to keep your hands off the cardio machine. Here are four specific reasons why:

1. Lower calorie burn. It's been estimated that you will burn 20 to 25 percent fewer calories if you hold onto cardio machines while working out. Furthermore, when you hold on, the digital calories-burned readout on the machine's console will be totally off because the machine doesn't know (or care) that you've been holding onto it.

2. Intensity negated. While adding resistance or an incline does increase intensity, holding onto cardio machines allows you to more comfortably lean back or forward, which totally negates the benefit of adding the resistance or incline in the first place. You think you're working harder. It definitely feels like you're working harder, but you're not. Basically you've attempted to ramp up your workout, but the net effect of holding onto the machine will be as if there's no resistance or incline at all. And using that same logic, it should now come as no surprise that the benefits of increasing the speed will also be largely negated if you simultaneously hold onto the machine while exercising.

3. Balance and coordination impaired. If you're not physically challenged in a way that requires support while moving from point A to point B, then you should not feel the need to support yourself while exercising on a treadmill, elliptical or whatever. Think about it—in your everyday life, do you feel the need to hold onto something when walking, jogging or running? I'm guessing no. And since this is the case, you'll need to carry over that same level of coordination while on the cardio machines. Furthermore, holding on throws off your body's natural gait, balance and sense of coordination, which is totally contrary to what you'd want to do when trying to get in shape.

4. Injury more likely. In my opinion, this is the biggest reason why you should take a hands-off approach to cardio machines. For example, most people think they're safer on the treadmill if they hold on. And I suppose this could be true if you're totally engrossed in Maury Povich's latest "You Are Not The Father" episode, and you need something to help brace yourself when you gasp at the paternity test results. But just recognize that by holding on, you're potentially setting yourself up for long-term injuries and pain. Shoulders, knees, the lower back and hips take the worst beating from the unnatural motion or gait that results from holding on. Here's a case in point:

> I know a woman in her late 20s with chronic shoulder pain and occasional tingling and numbness in her right arm. I would constantly see this woman at the gym holding on to the front of the treadmill while walking or running. One day, after learning that I was a physician, this woman asked me about her shoulder pain, why nothing was working to alleviate her pain, and if there was anything I could recommend to make it better. Now, I'm not a fan of doing curbside medical consultations, but in her case I made an exception and promptly let her know that her problem was most likely due to a pinched nerve and that her pain would almost certainly not get better if she kept holding onto to the treadmill. Furthermore, I told her that if she didn't stop with the treadmill-holding, her condition was likely to get worse. Just think about it: A relatively healthy woman in her late 20s dealing with a frustrating condition like chronic shoulder pain, so much so that she has difficulty resting her backpack on her shoulder for more than 10 minutes at a time. Plus she's got the added joy of now having to attend physical therapy and pay for pain meds. Sounds like tons of fun, huh? Don't say you weren't warned.

In conclusion, I'll repeat it once more for good measure: Hands off the cardio machines!

And if you absolutely feel the need to hold onto something to maintain your balance, I'd strongly advise cranking things down a bit—be it speed, intensity or incline—to a point where you're comfortable letting go and moving comfortably without support. Then as time goes on, you can gradually transition to higher speeds, intensities and inclines. You'll find that if you follow this tip, your body will adjust and you'll be able to support yourself just fine. Moreover, you'll have a safer and better workout.

MISTAKE 10
ALL CALORIES ARE CREATED EQUAL

YOU SAY: All calories are created equal.

I SAY: You may have heard this phrase before to prove the point that weight management is all about math. If you want to lose weight, create a caloric deficit. Generally, the magic number to lose one pound is considered to be about 3,500 calories. So according to the "all calories are created equal" theory, also known as the "a calorie is a calorie" doctrine, if you want to lose one pound in a week, you need to create a deficit of 3,500 calories over those seven days.

For the most part, that's true.

Problem is, the whole "all calories are created equal" statement is frequently taken a step further and used to argue that macronutrient proportions don't matter. According to this way of thinking, if you want to lose weight, simply maintain a caloric deficit. You can eat whatever proportions of fat, carbs or protein you want, and as long as you make sure to maintain a caloric deficit, you'll lose weight. All that matters is caloric deficit. Where calories come from is totally unimportant.

Whoops!

Now all that isn't entirely true.

Truth be told, macronutrient proportions matter very much with regards to not just weight loss, but also to overall health. Furthermore, which macronutrients your food calories originate from can ultimately affect how those calories are absorbed, as well as how efficiently those calories are metabolized and burned by your body.

The Thermic Effect

One of the chief factors that can change how your body uses a calorie is the macronutrient that brought that calorie into your body in the first place. Each macronutrient has a "cost" associated with breaking it down so that your body is able to use those calories for energy. This cost associated with breaking down macronutrients is called the "thermic effect of food" (TEF). The thermic effect of food is just a fancy name for the energy used up in the digestion, absorption and distribution of nutrients.

Generally speaking, fat is the easiest macronutrient to break down, costing the least amount of calories to metabolize. Carbs come next, while proteins are by far the most expensive source of fuel for your body to use. What this ultimately means is that a 2,500-calorie-per-day, high-protein diet actually adds *fewer* calories to the body than would a 2,500-calorie-per-day, high-carb diet or a 2,500-calorie-per-day, high-fat diet. I know that all this sounds weird, but it's scientifically proven. Because, truth be told, all calories are not created equal.

Protein

When it comes to protein, it's also worth noting that protein has been shown to have a significant impact on appetite. Specifically, and impressively, it decreases appetite. This means that if you increase your daily protein intake, you'll end up putting yourself at a dietary advantage. Namely, you'll be less likely to experience hunger and more likely to reduce your total calorie intake without even trying.

So a person who consciously increases his or her daily protein intake without making any conscious attempt to eat less is still likely to eat less anyway due to reduced appetite. This fact is another important example of how protein, carbohydrate and fat calories are not all created equal.

This protein-appetite correlation was demonstrated by a University of Washington School of Medicine study in which 19 subjects spent time on three different diets. First, the subjects followed a low-protein calorie maintenance diet for two weeks. After that, they switched to a high-protein diet with the same number of total calories for another two weeks. In the final stage, which lasted 12 weeks, the volunteers used the same high-protein diet. However, in the last 12 weeks, subjects had no calorie restrictions and were allowed to eat as much or as little as they wanted.

At the conclusion of the study, researchers reported that when subjects switched from the low-protein weight maintenance diet to the high-protein weight maintenance diet, they started feeling much fuller despite the fact that they were consuming the same number of calories. And even more amazing, during the unrestricted high-protein diet phase, subjects started to *voluntarily* reduce their daily caloric intake by 441 calories per day and lost almost 11 pounds, including more than eight pounds of body fat, on average.

Fiber

Although it's not a macronutrient, fiber is another component of food that can have a powerful and positive impact on weight loss. Technically speaking, dietary fiber is a type of carbohydrate, but fiber is unique in that it can't be digested or absorbed by the body. Ultimately, fiber won't contribute additional calories when eaten. In addition, when eaten, fiber will actually contribute to satiety despite not contributing additional calories. Consequently, a 100-calorie high-fiber food will reduce appetite more than a 100-calorie low-fiber food. Likewise, a person who increases his daily fiber consumption without making any conscious effort to eat less will wind up eating less anyway due to reduced appetite. As an added benefit, high-fiber foods can also improve your digestion and cholesterol profile. This all goes to show that overall, a calorie inside a high-fiber food is not equal to a calorie inside a low-fiber food. Yet another reason why all calories are not created equal.

Calorie Restriction and Metabolism

It's pretty much standard that when people are trying to lose weight, they'll drop their daily caloric intake. For example, if you decide to cut your daily energy intake by 500 calories (as based on the 3,500-calorie rule cited earlier), you can figure that you'll lose approximately a pound a week (500 calories/day x 7 days = 3,500 calories). Problem is, as time goes on, you'll most likely find that the 500-calorie deficit you created will no longer give you the one pound per week weight loss each subsequent week. And some weeks you may not lose any weight at all.

Huh?! How could that happen?

Here's what's going on:

Simply put, your body is very smart, and the fewer calories you consume, the fewer calories your body will want to burn. This phenomenon is believed to represent a metabolic adaptation wherein your body will essentially drop its metabolic rate and hold on tighter to the reduced number of calories you're eating, all in a very strategic effort to prevent caloric waste and subsequent starvation.

Moreover, from your body's perspective, that frustrating fatty tissue you're desperately trying to get rid of is in fact a special reserve for times of food scarcity or starvation. So when you start to limit your calorie intake in an effort to lose fat, your body will make some adjustments of its own to reduce your metabolic rate, reduce calorie burn, and hold onto body fat.

In fact, several long-term studies have found that following restricted calorie diets for long periods of time (months to years) resulted in a **significant reduction** in basal metabolic rates..

But even more profound is the effect that caloric deficits can have on elite athletes, even over a relatively short period of time. One study measured the metabolic activity in female athletes over the course of a single day and compared that to their body composition, with startling results. The female athletes who allowed themselves to hit several small caloric deficits during the day had more body fat and less muscle than those who distributed their meals more evenly throughout the day. In other words, this study found that you're more likely to have a leaner appearance and a better-looking body composition overall if you can match your caloric intake with your caloric needs, rather than letting your body think it needs to hold onto body fat because you're being stingy with caloric intake.

The Final Consensus on Calories

Wait a minute! I thought weight loss basically boiled down to calories in versus calories out, and creating a caloric deficit. That's what everyone is constantly saying.

Now you're telling me that all this isn't true?!

No, what I'm saying is that all calories are not created equal, and caloric deficit is just part of the *entire* weight loss equation.

Truth be told, the entire weight loss equation is very, very complex. For example, the weight loss equation you've been taught to follow looks like this:

Weight loss = Fewer calories in − More calories out

In reality, the real weight loss equation probably looks more like this:

$$\int_p^\infty \exp\left(-\pi^2 \frac{k^2}{L^2}\alpha\delta\right) dk = \int_0^\infty \exp\left(-\pi^2 \frac{k^2}{L^2}\alpha\delta\right) dk - \int_0^p \exp\left(-\pi^2 \frac{k^2}{L^2}\right.$$

$$= \frac{L\sqrt{\pi}}{2\pi\sqrt{\alpha\delta}} - \frac{L\sqrt{\pi}}{2\pi\sqrt{\alpha\delta}} \operatorname{erf}\left(\frac{\pi\sqrt{\alpha\delta}p}{L}\right) \cong$$

$$\cong \frac{L\sqrt{\pi}}{2\pi\sqrt{\alpha\delta}} - \frac{L\sqrt{\pi}}{2\pi\sqrt{\alpha\delta}}\left(1 - \frac{e^{-\pi^2 p^2\alpha\delta/L^2}}{\sqrt{\pi}\pi\sqrt{\alpha\delta}\frac{p}{L}}\left[1 - \frac{2!}{1!\left(2\pi\sqrt{\alpha\delta}\frac{p}{L}\right)^2} + \frac{4!}{2!\left(2\pi\sqrt{\alpha\delta}\frac{p}{L}\right)^4} - \right.\right.$$

$$\cong \frac{e^{-\pi^2 p^2\alpha\delta/L^2}}{2\pi^2 \frac{p}{L^2}\alpha\delta}\left[1 - \frac{2!}{1!\left(2\pi\sqrt{\alpha\delta}\frac{p}{L}\right)^2} + \frac{4!}{2!\left(2\pi\sqrt{\alpha\delta}\frac{p}{L}\right)^4} - \dots\right]$$

$$\frac{e^{-\pi^2 p^2\alpha\delta/L^2}}{2\pi^2 \frac{p}{L^2}\alpha\delta} < \frac{e^{-\pi^2 p^2\alpha\delta/L^2}}{\pi^2 \frac{p}{L^2}\alpha\delta}, \quad \frac{p^2\alpha\delta}{L^2} > 0.05$$

Quite frankly, most health and fitness experts know full well about the complexity of the factors that go into losing weight. Thing is, we don't get into the fine details of the entire equation because honestly, if we did get into it, the average person's head would probably explode.

So we experts keep it simple for the average person so you don't get overwhelmed with the minute details. In other words, we want you to focus on the big picture, not every single pixel in the image. Because yes, the "calories in versus calories out" model does work. It's just not all there is to losing weight.

Take elite athletes, for example. When it comes to elite athletes, trust and believe that their nutritional and training protocol does not begin and end with the "calories in versus calories out" model. Furthermore, the whole "all calories are created equal" statement is flat-out laughed off as a complete joke within the world of sports medicine and exercise science. Elite athletes are on a whole other level when it comes to fitness, performance, nutrition, and so on. So when elite athletes need to drop body fat, build muscle or even maintain a healthy weight, they're going to take many more factors into consideration, including meal timing, meal frequency and macronutrient ratios, and not just focus on "calories in versus calories out."

This point was demonstrated by a Japanese study in which boxers who were placed on a six-meals-a-day, weight-control diet lowered their body fat percentage *significantly* more than boxers who ate *exactly* the same number of calories in just two meals.

But how could these results be?

Clearly, if it's only about calories in versus calories out, both groups of boxers should have lost the same amount of weight. But they didn't, and it's because weight loss can be a lot more complex than calories in versus calories out.

All this said, the very basic principle of creating a caloric deficit to lose weight is indeed true. This was famously demonstrated when Mark Haub, a nutrition professor at Kansas State University, lost 27 pounds in 10 weeks on his infamous "Twinkie Diet." On this diet, Haub ate nothing but Twinkies and other highly processed junk foods. He also restricted his daily caloric intake to 1,800 calories. And to the astonishment of many, Haub lost weight. Twenty-seven pounds in 10 weeks to be exact! When you think about it, that's pretty darn good when compared to the average dieter.

Now, I'm not by any means encouraging you to start stuffing your face with Twinkies while maintaining a caloric deficit to lose weight. I'm just illustrating the point that caloric deficit does work even when you eat junk food. Of course, it should be noted that even Haub doesn't suggest following such a diet for other health reasons. Because while you could certainly lose weight with the "Twinkie Diet" or a diet similar to it, your general health would also most definitely take a nosedive.

Bottom line: Counting calories and creating a caloric deficit is definitely a useful weight loss strategy. So for the general purpose of weight loss, focus on creating a caloric deficit (which does assume that all calories are created equal). But while using a caloric deficit to lose weight, you should also keep in the back of your mind that the story doesn't end there.

And if you really want to be a rock star and step your fitness up to more of an elite level, recognize that you'll need to focus on more than just caloric deficit. If weight loss is your goal, look into adjusting your macronutrient ratios to include greater proportions of protein and fiber (while still creating a caloric deficit). Remember what I mentioned about elite athletes: They don't look at all calories as being the same. So if you aspire to have the body of an athlete, learn to think like an athlete. Ultimately, all calories are not created equal, and the way that a calorie affects your metabolism very strongly depends on where it originally came from.

MISTAKE 11
YOU SHOULD ALWAYS STRETCH BEFORE A WORKOUT

YOU SAY: You should always stretch before a workout.

I SAY: Since your elementary school gym class, you've been told to stretch before exercise. As a child, you probably gleefully went through the motions as your gym teacher, Coach Jockitch, instructed you through a range of stretching exercises like side bends and toe touches to prevent injury and improve performance. Now as an adult, if you're like most people, you probably skip the stretch and go right to your workout. Still, occasionally you might feel a small twinge of apprehension about whether *not* stretching could lead to injury down the road. So, is there any real merit to the stretching ritual?

First, before I answer that question, it would be best to differentiate between two types of stretching: static stretching and dynamic stretching. As the name suggests, static stretches are those in which you maintain a specific position for 20 to 30 seconds. Think things like touching your toes or a quadriceps stretch.

Dynamic stretching, on the other hand, focuses on movements that target a more fluid range of motion. Dynamic stretches could consist of a series of air squats, side lunges or other more fluid movements to help your body warm up. Other examples of dynamic stretches are arm circles, butt kicks and high knees. Basically, static stretching involves holding a pose for a set period of time, while dynamic stretching means more movement and something a little more exciting, or dynamic!

In general, static stretches are the type of stretching that most people do and think they should be doing before every workout. Therefore, static stretching is what we'll address here.

As far as modern exercise science is concerned, experts are pretty much unanimous in their disagreement that you should always stretch (that is, static stretch) before working out. In fact, studies have shown that static stretching may leave you worse off than if you didn't stretch at all. I'm sure many of you are in total shock right now at what I'm saying, mouths agape, wondering how I could go against the advice of your beloved Coach Jockitch. But let's take a moment to pick your jaw up off the floor and review the facts, and you'll see why static stretching before, and even after, every workout will not prevent injury or improve performance.

Injury Prevention

No one wants to get hurt when they're trying to get in shape, so it makes perfect sense to spend a little extra time stretching before a workout to protect yourself and prevent injury. I mean, that's what you've been taught by most personal trainers and fitness professionals.

Problem is, static stretching isn't going to protect you from injury.

Three different meta-analyses, which are essentially large reviews where experts compare the findings of many similar studies, looked into the actual benefits of static stretching, and all came up with the same result: Static stretching does nothing to prevent exercise injury.

Now, there's no doubt that static stretching increases flexibility and elongates muscles. But unless your goal is *just* to improve flexibility, it's best to avoid static stretching as part of your warm-up to prevent injury. In fact, some sports medicine specialists believe that static stretching could actually *increase* the risk of injury. This hypothesis is based on the fact that static stretching can cause small tears in muscle fibers, as well as have a pain-dulling (i.e., analgesic) effect on muscles. All in all, it's probably not a good idea to damage a muscle, increase your tolerance for pain, and then strenuously exercise that very same muscle.

Reduced Strength and Speed

Even worse, there's substantial research suggesting that static stretching could actually make you weaker and slower.

One very telling study took a group of 17 volunteers and had some perform 10 minutes of stretching, while the others did nothing for a warm-up. All of the subjects were then asked to perform jump squats for which their jump height, power and speed were all measured. The results showed that the group that stretched beforehand couldn't jump as high or as fast as the group that hadn't stretched.

This decline in performance with static stretching was also found in runners. In 2008, researchers at Louisiana State University decided to test out the effects of static stretching on exercise performance by enlisting the help of 19 particularly gifted sprinters. The sprinters were asked to warm up and then perform a 40-meter sprint, both with and without static stretches in their warm-up. Shockingly, the sprinters that stretched lost a full tenth of a second on their time, slowing down most significantly in the last half of the run. Similar results were found in a Miami University study that tested 18 sprinters over 100 meters; the study subsequently reported that pre-run static stretches caused a "significant slowing in performance ... in the second 20 (20-40) m of the [100 m] sprint trials."

Muscle Soreness and Recovery

Another reason people perform static stretches, particularly at the end of their workouts, is to reduce muscle soreness and improve speed of exercise recovery. This practice came about based on the old idea that delayed-onset muscle soreness (DOMS) was a result of spasms in the damaged muscle that ultimately restricted blood flow and caused pain. Since static stretching reduced spasms, it was concluded that static stretching could also be used to prevent and treat DOMS.

The problem is that in 1986, the spasm theory of DOMS was debunked. For some reason though, static stretching is still considered a useful treatment, despite an abundance of evidence proving that stretching does not help with the recovery of DOMS. In fact, a 2008 meta-analysis looked at 10 different studies and found conclusively that static stretching does nothing to reduce DOMS. And yet another study found that stretching was useless, not only in the case of DOMS, but also in post-exercise recovery as a whole.

The Smart Way to Stretch

So basically, all the research points to a simple conclusion: Static stretching before you exercise is useless and is, in some cases, a pretty bad idea. But does that mean that you should never stretch?

Of course not!

As mentioned earlier, static stretching is great for improving flexibility. While it's often overlooked when placed side by side with strength and endurance, flexibility is considered by many health authorities to be a benchmark of fitness. Having limber, flexible joints and muscles can go a long way toward preventing injury from accidents like slipping and falling. Static stretching is also especially useful when you do it *after* your muscles are warmed up, like after your workout, for example.

You might remember though, that at the outset of this discussion, I mentioned another form of stretch: dynamic stretching. Unlike static stretching, dynamic stretching has indeed been proven to increase muscular performance, agility, vertical jump and speed, while also preventing injury and encouraging recovery. So the next time you're prepping for a workout, skip the old Coach Jockitch routine of stretching, and instead of boring toe touches, get moving with air squats, side lunges, arm circles, butt kicks, high knees and other more fluid movements to help your body better stretch and warm up.

MISTAKE 12
FASTING KILLS METABOLISM AND PUTS YOUR BODY IN STARVATION MODE

YOU SAY: Fasting kills metabolism and puts your body in starvation mode.

I SAY: You've probably been cautioned against fasting by well-meaning friends, fitness gurus, and maybe even a few respected health professionals. They've told you that skipping meals could actually make it harder for you to lose weight. When you've mentioned an interest in fasting, they've thrown warnings at you like:

Your body will panic!

Your metabolism will screech to a halt and you'll stop burning fat!

Once you stop the fast and start eating, your body will increase the rate at which it stores fat!

While these warnings do initially *seem* like sensible adaptations that the body would make in times when food is scarce, all this hate against fasting is totally unfounded.

How so?

Although starvation mode is indeed a process that the body goes through to protect us from famine or times when food is otherwise unavailable, starvation mode simply doesn't happen when you just skip breakfast, dinner, or even a whole day's worth of meals.

In fact, to get a better understanding of the starvation process, researchers at the University of Rochester devised a study aimed at finding the precise time that it does take for our bodies to actually enter starvation mode. To do this, researchers closely observed humans and lab animals under very controlled conditions to see when this supposed wane in metabolism and "starvation mode" would actually kick in.

Can you guess how long it took?

Well, it definitely wasn't immediate. In the study, researchers waited—and waited, and waited—and finally, after *60 hours* it happened. But the decline in metabolic rate wasn't even that bad. On average, the subjects only experienced an eight percent decrease in metabolic activity. Not at all significant. Surprisingly enough, subsequent and similar research has actually found that a short fast (lasting from 36 to 48 hours) can actually cause a significant *boost* in metabolism. Now those results were totally unexpected!

True Starvation

In these early stages of food restriction, before true "starvation" begins, your body will use and begin to exhaust its stores of glycogen (i.e., carbohydrates) and fat as fuel. Glycogen and fat are the body's preferred sources of energy.

Now keep in mind, at this point, your stomach may be grumbling and you may *feel* like you're going to die if you don't eat something, but your body is actually doing just fine. Whether you realize it or not, your body has plenty of glycogen and fat stored up to function even though your stomach is empty and literally begging for satisfaction.

Also, during the early stages of food deprivation, your body will go through various steps to prepare itself, many of which are extremely beneficial. We'll talk more about these benefits a little later. Suffice it to say, it's not until after your body has almost completely exhausted its glycogen and fat stores that you'll actually enter starvation mode. This is the point when, since it has nothing else left to use, your body turns to its next available source of fuel—protein. Unfortunately, in our bodies, protein is primarily stored in the form of muscle, which is definitely something you don't want to break down for energy.

If starvation progresses and muscle starts being consumed for energy, you will subsequently become weaker, and your metabolic rate will begin to decline. At this point, your immune system will also start to shut down, making you more susceptible to disease. If starvation persists, eventually your vital organ systems will start to shut down, and in most starvation-related deaths, the ultimate cause of death will be heart failure.

Make no mistake, starvation is indeed a medical emergency. But as I mentioned earlier, it typically takes three days for this process to even *begin*. And furthermore, as you will soon learn, temporary, controlled fasts are not something to be feared because research has indeed shown that there are several benefits to restricting food for intermittent periods of time.

The Benefits

When your body starts to sense that its fat and glycogen stores are getting low, it's going to send signals to the brain that are simply designed to encourage you to go get some food. Adrenaline and noradrenaline are two chemical messengers that our brain releases to encourage us to go on the hunt for grub. I'm sure most of you immediately recognize the word "adrenaline" as something that makes you want to get up and go. And that is precisely what adrenaline and noradrenaline will work to do. Both of these hormones trigger increased mental focus, faster muscle contractions and increased metabolism.

All these changes are meant to increase our overall energy level and desire to go look for food. But for those of us who understand that our bodies aren't actually starving, timing exercise with the physiological changes that occur with increased adrenaline and noradrenaline can give us the perfect window to exploit things a bit in our favor. In other words, this window of sharper mental focus, faster muscle contractions and increased metabolism is a great time to schedule a workout because you'll be more likely to perform better than usual and thus burn more calories.

As more studies are carried out on fasting, more benefits are steadily being revealed that can be further exploited and used to our advantage. For example, it was also found that fasts generally lasting from 16 to 24 hours can increase insulin sensitivity, fat metabolism, resistance to disease and even your overall lifespan. Granted, we don't completely understand all the mechanisms at work here, but the benefits are clear and well-substantiated. Altogether this means that you can most certainly fast for intermittent periods of time without worrying that your body will enter starvation mode and eventually waste away to nothing.

Intermittent Fasting

A nutritional strategy that capitalizes on the benefits of fasting, known as intermittent fasting (IF), has become quite popular. Generally speaking, intermittent fasting involves splitting your day into "fasting" and "feeding" periods. A common IF approach is the 16/8 split. This means that you would pack all of your calories for the day into an eight-hour window. For example, if your first meal is at 9 a.m., your last would be at 5 p.m. The 16/8 split is just one iteration of the intermittent fasting protocol, and there are many others, like the 20/4 split.

I won't get deep into the specifics of intermittent fasting, and I just wanted to briefly mention it here as a viable fasting option for the curious-minded. Intermittent fasting carries the same overall health benefits I mentioned earlier, and intermittent fasting is something I practice regularly, though not daily. Currently, I perform an intermittent fast one day per week, typically on a Sunday, and without question, I believe intermittent fasting has helped to improve my fitness gains tremendously, as well as made my nutrition much easier to manage.

If you're curious about fasting in general, or intermittent fasting specifically, I'd suggest doing a bit more research on these topics and giving it a shot. There are so many fasting options with tons of research behind them, all with various benefits, including increased growth hormone levels and improved insulin sensitivity, to name a few. The key thing to remember is that fasting, despite some of its negative press, does have its place in a healthy lifestyle. Not only will it give you a massive boost towards your fitness goals, but it can even improve your overall health.

MISTAKE 13

YOU CAN "SPOT REDUCE" BODY FAT WITH SPECIFIC EXERCISES

YOU SAY: You can "spot reduce" body fat with specific exercises.

I SAY: Before I explain why "spot reduction" doesn't work, let me explain what spot training is. Spot training, sometimes called spot reduction, is the idea that you can target and remove fat from just one area of the body without affecting the shape of surrounding body parts. Spot training is one of the most persistent fitness myths out there, and it just refuses to die thanks to late-night infomercials pimping half-baked exercise equipment and supplements.

The spot reduction myth is especially pervasive at gyms, and people frequently ask fitness professionals like myself what exercises they can do or what machine they should use to spot reduce. For example, when women make statements like, "I want to lose weight *here*, but I don't want to lose my butt," that is a form of desired spot reduction.

So is spot reduction possible?

No.

And yes, while people can and do lose weight in certain areas of the body when they work out—some areas more and faster than others—

in general, you can't just specifically "target" a body part for fat loss. Sorry, it's just not possible. Not because *I* say so, but because *your body* says so.

How We Gain and Lose Fat

Simply put, the same way you don't get to decide where that fat goes when it comes in is the same way you don't get to tell it how or when to leave. The only way to lose weight from one area—for example, your stomach—is to lose weight *everywhere*. And the most efficient way to burn that fat from everywhere is through a combination of cardiovascular exercise, strength training and a healthy diet.

To make things even more complicated, everyone gains and/or loses fat differently. For you, the stomach area might be a main trouble spot, or maybe your arms. For most men, the most stubborn area for fat loss will be with their stomach while women fight against the stubborn fat trifecta: the stomach, thighs and butt.

This means that if your stomach is your main target, you have to keep losing overall body fat until your body decides that it's good and ready to let go of that pesky belly fat. And sorry, all the twists and crunches in the world won't speed up the process.

In fact, a study published in *The Journal of Strength and Conditioning Research* proved this very point when researchers found that abdominal exercise did absolutely nothing to reduce abdominal fat. Arguably the most compelling evidence refuting the myth of spot reduction, this study was conducted at the University of Massachusetts in the mid-1980s. In this investigation, participants had to do a vigorous abdominal exercise training program that consisted of 5,000 sit-ups over the course of 27 days. At the end of the training program, fat biopsies were taken from each participant's abdomen, buttocks and upper back. And contrary to what spot-reducing proponents would have you believe, the results of the study revealed that fat decreased similarly at *all* three sites—not just in the abdominal region.

Another interesting study found that in professional tennis players, both their dominant (i.e., swinging) arm and non-dominant arm contained the same amount of fat. It might sound a little ridiculous that someone actually took the time to measure fat in the arms of professional tennis players, but these findings further support the fallacy of the spot training myth, because if spot training were indeed possible, it would be most evident in professional tennis players who spend an inordinate amount of time exercising their dominant arms. As expected, in those tennis players, the dominant arm was slightly bigger in circumference due to more developed muscles. But the difference in body fat between their dominant and non-dominant arm was negligible.

How to Stay Fat-Loss Focused

In your battle against the bulge, there are a few things to remember, particularly to keep yourself sane and motivated.

First, as noted, there are some areas where your body will resist burning off its fat. Unfortunately, in most people it's the area that they're obsessed with the most—the stomach. Thing is, you'll just need to be patient and not get discouraged. Keep exercising and the weight will come off. Again, patience is key. As badly as you may want those love handles gone, just remember that your body will hold onto those handles until it's good and ready to let go.

Second, don't pay too much attention to the scale. It's not uncommon for people to lose a good deal of body fat while not noticing much difference on the scale. This is especially true with strength training. In fact, when lifting weights, it is possible to lose body fat but actually see your weight go *up.* This kooky phenomenon is due to the dense weight of muscle gained.

Third, if you really want to track fat loss accurately, I'd suggest periodically getting your body fat tested with body fat calipers. You can get this done by a professional or you can buy body fat calipers and test yourself. Body fat calipers cost anywhere from $5 to upwards of $80. I usually tell newbies to hop on Amazon and invest in a $5 pair of calipers. Body fat calipers are relatively easy to use (read the instructions thoroughly!) and when used properly, calipers will give you a very good idea of the fat loss progress you're making.

Last but not least, another great way to "measure" your progress is to just keep it simple and focus on the obvious. How do your clothes fit? It takes less than five seconds to throw on your favorite t-shirt or pair of skinny jeans to assess how much your body is changing. Also, consider keeping a picture diary of yourself. Let me tell you, the camera doesn't lie, and keeping a diary of pics is a great way to keep yourself motivated because you'll actually *see* the transformation in full effect.

MISTAKE 14
DON'T EAT LATE AT NIGHT IF YOU WANT TO LOSE WEIGHT

YOU SAY: Don't eat late at night if you want to lose weight.

I SAY: Ever had that fear of eating past 9 p.m. because you thought you'd get fat? You're not alone.

The whole "eat late, gain weight" myth has been around for years, and although some people could swear that their late-night eating habits do make them gain weight, numerous studies have consistently shown that nighttime eating does not actually cause weight gain if you stay within your body's daily caloric needs.

Moreover, the British Medical Journal recently put the late-night eating myth to bed in an article in which they reviewed the results of various studies on the topic of nighttime eating and weight gain. After looking at countless clinical studies throughout the world, they found no link between eating at night and weight gain. In addition, the American Dietetic Association agrees that when it comes to weight gain, it's not about the timing but rather the amount being eaten.

But It Happened to Me!

Where many people get into trouble with eating late at night is that they binge and subsequently take in more calories than they need in a day. This is often the case when people practice poor eating habits and/or put themselves on extreme diets where they take in too few calories during the day. As a result, these folks end up feeling ravenous at night and consequently fall victim to stuffing their faces with junk food.

Another reason people who eat late at night can end up gaining weight is that they are "mindlessly eating" while sitting in front of the television or computer. Interestingly enough, people who mindlessly eat aren't truly hungry but rather are eating out of habit, boredom, stress or fatigue. People also tend to make poor food choices when they mindlessly eat, regardless of the time of day. Cookies, chips, leftover pizza, ice cream, desserts and other sugar-filled processed foods are often first dibs. Consuming these foods leads to racking up more calories than the body needs, resulting in weight gain.

In reality, the actual problem wasn't **when** food was eaten, but rather **the type and amount** of food eaten.

In addition, while many people will swear up and down that they can miraculously lose weight when they stop eating late, this weight loss is often due to the fact that these same people simply have stopped eating the same junk they used to at night. In essence, they start becoming more self-aware and more cognizant of the importance of meal planning. They begin making better food choices during the day, so they're not as hungry and likely to gorge at night.

Time Is Not a Factor

Weight loss boils down to a bit of biochemistry and simple mathematics. Simply put, if you keep your insulin in check (that is, if don't consume a lot of sugars and processed carbs), while also making sure the amount of calories you eat is less than the amount you burn, you will lose weight. Conversely, if you regularly eat foods that spike insulin (like sugars and processed carbs), which stimulates fat storage, while also eating more calories than you burn, you will gain weight. It's that simple, folks. Meal timing doesn't really matter. Remember, your body will only store calories as fat if you take in more calories than you burn in a day, regardless of the time of day you choose to consume those excess calories.

For those who need help making better food choices and practicing better eating habits, I recommend these tips to help control total daily calorie intake:

- Eat a protein-rich breakfast

- Eat protein and fiber with every meal

- Drink a glass of water before each meal

- Avoid eating while multitasking

- Eat at the dining room or kitchen table instead of in front of the TV or computer

Also, I know some of you may have heard reputable health and fitness experts advise not eating after a certain hour of the day. But I want to point out that these experts make this suggestion not because they believe your body processes food differently at night. Instead, some experts give the "don't eat late" speech because they understand basic psychology and realize that setting a time beyond which you cannot eat will ultimately reduce the likelihood of you snacking on calorie-laden foods, which in turn will reduce your total calorie input for the day.

Bottom line: When all is said and done, feel free to eat at whatever time is most convenient for you with no worries about the impact it will have on your weight. If you want to lose weight, you should be worried about insulin regulation and total calorie consumption—not whether you can cram in your last meal by 8:59 p.m.

MISTAKE 15
WHEN DOING CARDIO, YOU WANT YOUR HEART RATE IN THE "FAT-BURNING" ZONE

YOU SAY: When doing cardio, you want your heart rate in the "fat-burning zone."

I SAY: In gyms all over the world, there exists an idea that if you want to burn fat effectively during cardio, you will need to maintain your heart rate in a very specific zone. Fancy, color-coded charts decorate treadmills, bikes and ellipticals to show you exactly where your heart rate should be in order to melt fat away. You can also calculate this magical heart rate by subtracting your age from 200 and multiplying this number by 0.6. If you consciously keep your heart rate at this number while exercising, so the story goes, you'll be in the "fat-burning zone." Some machines even do all the work for you, figuring out your target zone and keeping you there by monitoring your pulse and adjusting the difficulty of your workout as needed.

What has given this myth a degree of scientific legitimacy, and has thus made it especially difficult to uproot, is the fact that this myth is based on a small amount of truth.

The truth has its basis in the observation that that low-intensity exercise like walking does indeed tap mainly into fat stores, whereas higher intensity activities like running or sprinting will pull much more heavily from carbohydrate stores. Therein lies the origin of this theory: If you keep your heart rate in the "fat-burning zone," which is roughly 55 to 65 percent of your maximum heart rate, then you will burn more fat than if you exercised at higher levels of intensity.

In a nutshell: If you exercise at a *lower* intensity, you'll burn *more* fat.

Sounds pretty sweet, huh?

Why work harder, when you can take it easy and burn more fat, right?

This, my friends, is why the fat-burning zone myth is so attractive. However, truth is that the whole "fat-burning zone" idea is a total bust. Let's take a closer look at two specific reasons this is so.

Reason #1: The Fat-Burning Zone Confuses Absolute versus Relative Fat Burn

To understand the fat-burning zone myth, you need to understand how your body uses energy during exercise. Simply put, during exercise your body draws energy primarily from two places: fat stores and glycogen stores. Fat is stored in fat cells. Glycogen is the storage form of carbohydrates and is stored in your muscles and liver.

The fat-burning zone was conceived because, at lower exercise intensities, more fat is burned relative to glycogen. As I mentioned earlier, low-intensity exercise like walking does indeed tap mainly into fat stores. Moreover, if you keep the intensity low and exercise at 50 percent of your max heart rate, your body will burn a ratio of 60 percent fat to 40 percent glycogen. At 75 percent of your max heart rate, the burn ratio becomes 35 percent to 65 percent, and at higher intensities, the burn ratio is even lower and tilts even more in favor of glycogen.

Isn't this awesome?!

Basically, you can just stroll around the block (as oppose to doing heavy sprints) and actually lose a lot more fat!

I hope you're starting to smell something fishy with this idea of a fat-burning zone.

So why the heck would I tell you the "fat-burning zone" is a mistake and advise you to exercise more intensely if you'll just end up burning less fat?

The reason why is because it's all about *total* calories. Simply put, low-intensity workouts burn fewer *total calories*. And those *total* calories are what really matter, especially when you take the time factor into consideration.

Here's an example to better illustrate the point:

> Say you have two groups exercise for 30 minutes, with one group doing a low-intensity workout while the other does a high-intensity workout. In that 30 minutes' time, the high-intensity group will likely burn double the calories as the low-intensity group. So let's say at the end of 30 minutes, the high-intensity group will clock in at a total 400 calories burned, versus the low-intensity group's total of 200 calories burned.

Now let's do some simple math here.

Knowing that the low-intensity group is exercising at 50 percent of max heart rate, that means of the 200 total calories burned, 60 percent of those calories will come from fat, or 120 fat calories. On the flip side, the high-intensity group would have exercised at 75 percent of max heart rate and burned a total of 400 calories; 35 percent of those calories would come from fat, or 140 fat calories.

So now you see how higher exercise intensity will burn more fat than lower exercise intensity (140 versus 120), even despite a smaller percentage of fat being burned through higher-intensity exercise. Moreover, the difference in fat burn between low- and high-intensity exercise becomes even more pronounced the more higher-intensity training sessions you substitute per week and the longer you exercise.

Reason #2: The Fat-Burning Zone Has No Afterburn Effect

When you exercise at low intensities, increased calorie burn pretty much comes to a halt the moment you stop exercising. However, when you exercise intensely, your body will undergo a sort of metabolic shift that enables it to actually continue burning calories at an increased rate even after the workout is completed. This really cool metabolic shift is known as the afterburn effect, or what my fellow brainiac sports specialists refer to as excess post-exercise oxygen consumption (EPOC).

It's important to note that the actual degree of the afterburn effect will vary by individual, exercise method, and exercise intensity. Still, the afterburn effect is very real and a very cool way to continue torching calories even after you're done exercising.

There are numerous studies that validate the afterburn effect, and in one landmark study at Appalachian State University in Boone, North Carolina, researchers recently found that the key to the extra calorie burn was not the length of the workout, but rather, the intensity.

In this landmark study, participants alternated between days of 45-minute sessions of vigorous exercise—intense enough that it was difficult to hold a conversation. To accurately monitor the minute-by-minute calorie burn, participants lived in a chamber that measured all their metabolic activity for 24-hour periods. Using advanced technology, researchers found that the days of intense exercise did produce a measurable caloric difference. Ultimately, it was found that in the 14 hours after the intense workout, participants burned an average of 190 extra calories. And though burning an extra 190 calories after just one intense workout session won't immediately cause a person to shed a ton of weight, make no mistake, this type of additional calorie burn does most certainly add up over time as you add more intense training sessions to your training protocol. Furthermore, for busy people, more intense workouts like interval training are substantially more efficient to help you burn more calories in much less time, and thus burn more fat overall.

High-Intensity Interval Training (HIIT)

One of the more popular trends in the fitness world right now is high-intensity interval training, or HIIT. This exercise trend has spread like wildfire because it torches more calories than low-intensity, steady-state cardio and takes less time than traditional low-intensity, steady-state cardio, while having the added bonus of preserving lean muscle mass. In addition to that, HIIT improves your insulin sensitivity, spikes your growth hormone levels and stimulates the body to release chemicals that suppress appetite. Several large studies have backed up these benefits of HIIT, and as mentioned earlier, HIIT has another added bonus—the afterburn effect. So with HIIT, not only will you burn more calories in less time, preserve your lean muscle mass, improve your insulin sensitivity, spike your growth hormone levels and lower your appetite, but you'll also keep your metabolism elevated and continue to burn off extra calories and fat even after you're done working out!

I know what you're thinking now: *WHERE CAN I SIGN UP?!*

Hands down, exercise science has shown that high-intensity training protocols like HIIT are a more effective weight loss method. Another thing that makes HIIT so useful is how easily it can be incorporated into a workout. For standard HIIT protocols you don't need any equipment, and there are also many interval protocols, so you can pick the one that fits you best and incorporate it into your running, cycling, swimming or even elliptical workout.

Here's a standard sample HIIT workout for outdoor running:

1. Start with a 2-3 minute brisk warm-up walk at a relatively low-to-moderate intensity

2. Now sprint as fast as you can for 30-60 seconds (*And when I say "sprint as fast as you can," I mean sprint like Channing Tatum is wearing see-through Speedos and waiting for you at the finish line!*)

3. Next, walk slowly for 1-2 minutes so you can catch your breath and recover

4. Repeat this cycle for a full 20-30 minutes

5. When you're done, allow yourself a 2-3 minute, low-intensity cool-down

And that's it! As you can see, HIIT is a very simple exercise protocol. Now, I didn't say it was *easy*, I said it was *easy to implement*. Yes, HIIT will and should kick your butt, but the rules are so simple that anyone can start doing HIIT. All this said, if torching fat is your main objective, your mission—should you choose to accept it—is to ignore the whole "fat-burning zone," up your exercise intensity, and get with the real deal—HIIT!

MISTAKE 16
TO LOSE WEIGHT, DRINK LOTS OF PROTEIN SHAKES AND EAT LOTS OF PROTEIN BARS

YOU SAY: To lose weight, drink lots of protein shakes and eat lots of protein bars.

I SAY: Preparing healthy, protein-rich meals everyday (or healthy meals in general) can be a bit time consuming, which is why protein supplements are often a must for hardcore athletes and fitness fanatics who know the important role protein plays in nutrition, performance and even weight loss.

The obvious benefit of using protein supplements is that they require very little prep time and are therefore easy, breezy "grab and go" meals. For example, a protein shake with 30 grams of protein will be a lot easier to scarf down than a thick, juicy steak. Protein supplements also require no refrigeration and are very portable. Last but not least, protein supplements can save you money, especially when you take into account that protein supplements cost less at 30 grams of protein per serving than foods like beef, salmon and other popular whole-food protein food sources. And let's face it, the extra cash saved from using protein supplements definitely comes in handy when you want to splurge on a new pair of Nikes.

Why You Need Adequate Protein in Your Diet

Here are a few of the numerous health benefits of protein:

Anabolism

Eating protein puts your body in an anabolic state. In terms of muscle building, "anabolism" refers to the construction, as opposed to the breakdown, of muscle tissue. The opposite of anabolism is catabolism, or the breakdown of tissue. Take for example, the process of burning fat. That is a catabolic process.

When it comes to exercise, one important thing to recognize is that regardless of the type of exercise, the body will break down some degree of muscle while it also works to break down or burn fat. This is especially true with very strenuous exercise of long duration. Therefore, it's very important to counteract the catabolic effects of exercise on muscle tissue with adequate protein intake.

Growth Hormone Regulation

Proper growth hormone levels are essential for good health. Growth hormone contains 190 amino acids, and eating enough protein ensures that your body has the necessary building blocks to construct growth hormone. Inadequate protein intake can and will ultimately lead to less growth hormone production, and growth hormone deficiency will ultimately result in issues like decreased metabolism, decreased bone density, muscle loss and numerous other health problems.

IGF-1 (Insulin-like growth factor 1)

IGF-1 allows muscle cells to properly respond to growth hormone. IGF-1 itself is a protein that contains over 70 amino acids, so without proper protein intake, IGF-1 levels will decrease, making it harder for your body to utilize available growth hormone.

Metabolism

Protein requires more energy to digest than fats and carbs, so eating an adequate amount of protein will inherently boost your metabolism. On the flip side, eating less-than-ideal amounts of protein can drop your metabolism, making it difficult for the body to burn fat.

Insulin

Hands down, insulin is the most important hormone in the fat-burning and muscle-building process. Simply put, if insulin is present in the blood beyond a certain threshold, the body will not (and cannot) burn fat. This is where protein becomes your fat-burning ally. Protein helps keep insulin levels low and stable, which is a critical requirement in the fat-burning process.

Who Can Benefit from Protein Supplements?

Pretty much anyone can benefit from protein supplements; typically, protein supplements are used by three categories of people for various reasons.

Bodybuilders

For those looking to add muscle mass, protein supplementation isn't an option—it's a requirement! Whether you're a whey protein addict or like to have a protein bar handy just in case, protein supplements are a bodybuilder's safety net.

Athletes

Protein supplementation isn't just for bodybuilders. Hard-training athletes need extra protein for energy, to repair muscle, and to ensure proper body functioning.

Dieters

Dieters can certainly benefit from protein-rich foods because they help speed up metabolism and fat burn. Protein also leaves you feeling more satisfied after a meal. Oftentimes dieters will use protein supplements simply to control daily calorie intake and fend off hunger.

Protein Supplements versus Whole Foods

A plethora of diet protein shakes floods the market—some great, some good, many not so good.

The question is: Do protein supplements work for weight loss?

Short answer: Yes, they can work. But only when chosen wisely *and* used wisely. It's very common to come across so-called "healthy protein supplements" that contain lots of fattening sugar and sweeteners like high-fructose corn syrup (which is often the case with cheap protein bars). In many cases you'll also come across so-called "healthy protein supplements" with vitamin and mineral profiles that are totally unbalanced and lack fiber, which is very important for keeping you satisfied and full during your diet.

In addition, in the case of protein bars versus whole foods like chicken or vegetables, a more compact protein bar will take up very little stomach volume, meaning you might get hungry again pretty soon. Furthermore, in regards to protein shakes, liquid calories are much easier to consume than whole foods, making it easier to over-consume calories. In fact, studies have shown that people consume 12 to 20 percent more calories when they have a liquid meal as opposed to eating a solid meal. Interestingly enough, the average American consumes about 1/3 of his or her calories in liquid form, which is one of the very reasons why the nation is facing this horrid obesity epidemic. *Hello, sodas and fruit smoothies!*

Now, I want to go on record that I am indeed a huge fan *and* advocate of protein supplements. But I'm very discriminating about which protein supplements I use and recommend. Furthermore, I don't rely solely on protein supplements for all my daily protein or nutritional needs. I believe the best nutrition comes from whole foods, and the majority of dietary protein should come from excellent protein food sources like meat, fish, poultry, eggs, cottage cheese and Greek yogurt.

The take-home from this information is that for the purposes of fat loss (or even muscle gain) protein supplements should be used as a *supplement* to a solid training and nutrition program. Last but not least, when it comes to the cost of protein supplements, I don't pinch pennies and I strongly advise that you don't either. Your goal should be to use the best-quality protein supplements, and ultimately I do believe that when it comes to protein supplements, you get what you pay for.

Protein Supplement Types

Before we get to my tips on how to pick a good protein powder, here is a quick protein primer of the most popular supplement types:

Whey Protein

Whey protein (also called "whey concentrate") makes up 20 percent of total milk protein. Whey is recognized for its excellent amino acid profile. Also, whey is a quick digesting protein. This means that when consumed, whey protein will start breaking down almost immediately to provide vital nutrients to your muscles.

Whey Protein Isolate

Most whey protein powders on store shelves are made up of bulk portions of whey concentrate and a small portion of whey isolate. A whey protein isolate source is one that has been chemically purified. In other words, whey protein isolate contains more protein, less fat and less lactose per serving. Typically, most whey protein isolates contain 90 to 98 percent protein, while whey concentrates contain 70 to 85 percent protein. For this reason, whey isolates (or protein isolates in general) are considered the "highest quality" proteins and are typically more expensive.

Casein Protein

Casein protein makes up 80 percent of total milk protein. Casein is also recognized for its excellent amino acid profile. However, casein is a slow digesting protein and will not start breaking down as quickly as whey. This can be a bad thing if quick recovery is your goal. But it can also be a good thing since slower-digesting proteins tend to help you stay fuller for longer.

Egg Protein Powder

Egg protein is often recognized as an excellent protein source since it has a complete profile of essential amino acids and branched-chain amino acids. However, one downside for some is that egg protein is sometimes harder to digest than other proteins and can leave you with a bloated, gassy feeling.

Vegan/Vegetarian Protein Powders

There are a few protein options out there for vegans and vegetarians. These protein powders are a great alternative for those with any allergies or food restrictions to gluten, yeast, milk, eggs, soy, nuts, and shellfish. Rice, hemp and pea protein powders are all complete proteins with decent nutritional profiles. Soy protein is also a very popular option. Derived from soybeans, soy powders make for an ideal alternative for those who do not consume animal products such as whey. While soy protein is high in branched-chain amino acids and digests quickly, it does mix poorly and is still viewed as a lower-quality protein alternative because the body cannot absorb it as well. Because of this, soy protein is not the most desirable protein source for those looking to build muscle.

Protein Blends

Protein blends are a combination of several types of protein. Why would you want a blend of proteins? Well, for one, protein combinations such as a whey-casein blend are a great way to tap into the benefits of consuming both fast-digesting and slow-digesting protein sources at the same time. Often, bodybuilders looking to exploit their full muscle-growth potential will use a blended protein powder. A blend can also be more cost effective then a pure protein isolate.

How to Pick a Healthy Protein Powder

Now let's move on to picking a healthy protein powder. In making this choice, I instruct folks to focus on these five factors:

1. Purpose of Powder

An important aspect to consider is the purpose of the protein powder. Since you're reading *And That's Why You're Fat*, we're going to assume you would like to lose weight. Getting enough protein in your diet is going to be crucial to keeping metabolism up, stimulating fat loss, preserving your precious lean muscle mass, and improving your health overall. For most women wanting to lose weight (and for those who don't have any special dietary restrictions), a standard whey protein powder will be sufficient for your needs. I consider whey protein isolates king among protein powders, and this is the type of protein supplement I primarily use. In fact, whether it comes to weight loss or muscle gain, hands down, whey protein is by far the most popular form of protein powder because of its amino acid profile and cost effectiveness.

2. Nutrition Facts and Ingredient List

When assessing a protein powder (or any food item for the matter) you should totally ignore the front of the package. I know, I know, the front of the package is usually so pretty and eye-catching. But that's how food manufacturers get you. So ignore the front. The nutritional info you really want to pay attention to is not on the front; it's on the back of the panel, which incidentally is the place few people read. Guys, I can't stress enough how important it is that you get in the habit of reading food labels. Don't just trust a food item because it has the word "HEALTHY" plastered all over the front label in bold lettering and glitter.

When assessing a protein powder, it's very simple: First, you want to check out the Nutrition Facts on the back label for calories per serving, and then you want to assess the macronutrient breakdown. The three macronutrients are: fat, carbohydrates and protein. I usually opt for a whey protein powder with 120 to 140 calories per scoop. I also look for those that are low fat (less than 2 grams of fat per serving), low sugar (zero to no more than 1 gram of sugar per serving) and high protein (more than 25 grams of protein per scoop).

The next thing I look at is the ingredient list, which is typically found below the Nutrition Facts. When you look at an ingredient list, keep in mind that the ingredients listed first are the most abundant. The lower on the list the ingredient, the less of it there is in the product. (This rule applies to regular foods as well). When examining the ingredient list, I try to find a product that doesn't have a laundry list of ingredients. As a general rule of thumb, I tend to gravitate to protein powders with no more than 10 to 12 ingredients. (Note: For protein blends, each type of protein is often listed, and I do not count each separate protein as a separate ingredient. I count all of the protein types together as one single ingredient.)

3. Amino Acid Profile

Amino acids are the building blocks of protein. The 20 amino acids found within proteins are separated into two categories: essential and non-essential amino acids. Essential amino acids cannot be created in the human body and must be obtained from food. Non-essential amino acids can be synthesized, or created, in the human body. There are nine essential amino acids. Since non-essential amino acids can be manufactured by the body, it's important to look for a protein powder with a good essential amino acid profile. Branched-chain amino acids, also called BCAAs, refer to a chain of the three essential amino acids: leucine, isoleucine and valine. These three essential amino acids make up over one-third of skeletal muscle in the body and play a vital role in protein synthesis. So when selecting a protein powder, you want to pay close attention to whether the protein supplement contains leucine, isoleucine and valine. You can also look into purchasing stand-alone branched-chain amino acid supplements.

4. Sugar and Sweetener Content

Protein powders will often contain sweeteners and flavoring agents, which is not exactly the definition of "clean" foods. Still, there are in fact many high-quality protein powders that also contain sweeteners. The short and sweet (no pun intended) is to look for powders that have 1 gram (or zero grams) of sugar per serving, and scan the ingredients list for added sweeteners like stevia (a natural sweetener) or sucralose (an artificial one). Honestly, I won't shun a protein powder just because it contains an artificial sweetener. I weigh things on a case-by-case basis. The choice is yours when it comes to artificial versus natural sweeteners. However, there is one type of sweetener I make no exception for in any protein supplement—high-fructose corn syrup (HFCS). If you see high-fructose corn syrup anywhere in the protein supplement ingredients, don't buy it!

5. Taste and Mixability

For many folks, this is really what it's all about—taste! And who doesn't want a protein powder that tastes good?! Protein powders really have come a long way, and many brands make a variety of flavors that taste delicious. The best way to find the right one for you is obviously to sample a few. Stores like Whole Foods and Vitamin Shoppe sell single serving-size samples, so try those. And don't forget to ask your friend if you can bum a taste of her protein powder.

As far as mixability, you're looking at two options: shaker or blender. Will you need to make a protein shake when you're already out and about? Or, do you plan to be at home, in the presence of your handy-dandy blender? For those of you who need to throw together a shake while you're on the go, I'd suggest picking up an easy mixing powder (whey isolates tend to be the best as far as mixability). You'll also need an efficient way to mix the powder, and I find that shaker bottles work well. They're about $10 and completely worth it if you want to avoid the unpleasant taste of unmixed, dry protein powder in your shake. That said, if you have a blender and the time to use it, mixability won't be much of an issue.

How to Pick a Healthy Protein Bar

Protein bars are quick and convenient, but not all protein bars are created equal. In fact, if you were to look at the nutrition facts of some popular protein bars, they would actually qualify more as candy bars than nutrition bars, which totally defeats the purpose if you're trying to eat healthy and lose weight. Below are six tips for picking a protein bar. (Note: When it comes to the fat and sugar requirements, apply these tips to protein powder selection as well.)

1. Calories versus Size of the Bar

If you're trying to lose weight, downing a small-sized 300-calorie protein bar isn't exactly going to make fat loss easy, especially if you've decided to limit your total calorie intake to, say, 1,200 calories a day. Think about it: That's 1/4 of your total daily calories in one bar that may not even fill you up for a few hours. So pay attention to the calories, as well as to the size of your protein bar.

2. Protein Source

As for the protein content, stick with bars that are made primarily from whey protein. If the first words on the ingredients list read things like "calcium caseinate" or "soy protein," I would not recommend buying, since those are inferior proteins. Also, if you are really trying to get the best protein bang for your buck and stave off hunger, I'd stick with bars that contain at least 16 grams of protein per serving.

3. Fat

Choose a bar that contains some fat since this will slow down the release of the carbs into the blood stream and make it more balanced overall. Just watch the total grams of fat, and totally avoid any bars that contain trans fat (aka "hydrogenated oils").

4. Sugar

Too much sugar in your diet will make you fat and keep you fat. Period. Overall, you need to be very mindful of your daily sugar intake, and personally, I won't touch a protein bar with more than 6 grams of sugar in it. Next, you want to avoid bars that contain high-fructose corn syrup (HFCS) in the ingredients. Also be mindful of bars that contain sugar alcohols like erythritol, sorbitol, maltitol and xylitol. Some manufacturers add sugar alcohols for sweetness but don't have to list it as a carbohydrate on the nutrition facts panel, making the claim that these sugar alcohols have no influence on blood sugar levels. But this is far from true.

For example, maltitol has a glycemic index (GI) of 52 (table sugar is 60). The glycemic index is a scale that ranks foods according to how much they raise blood sugar. Thus maltitol, as seen from its GI ranking, will raise your blood sugar significantly. As for calories, although maltitol does deliver only three calories per gram as opposed to sugar (which has four), maltitol does still add calories to your total daily calorie and carbohydrate intake. Another common sugar substitute sometimes added to protein bars (and protein powders) is maltodextrin, which is actually a glucose polymer. And while technically not a sugar, maltodextrin is something you may want to avoid in your protein supplements because it registers higher on the GI scale than a slice of white bread.

The key thing to remember about sugar and sugar substitutes is that while they don't look too terribly bad on the label, they can affect blood sugar levels, some more than others. An increase in blood sugar will in turn drive up your insulin levels, which will ultimately make weight loss very difficult.

5. Carbs-to-Protein Ratio

You always want be sure the protein content is higher than the carbs. The best scenario for fat loss will be, at a bare minimum, a 2:1 ratio of grams of protein to net carbs (net carbs = the total grams of carbs minus grams of fiber). Remember, the protein content is what makes a protein bar a "protein bar." So if there are more grams of carbs than protein, or even worse, more grams of sugar than protein, you definitely need to find another protein bar.

6. Fiber

Look for bars that contain at least 8 grams of fiber, and definitely more fiber than sugar. Fiber will help promote regularity, control blood sugar spikes, and help you feel full longer.

MISTAKE 17 THE MORE YOU SWEAT, THE MORE FAT YOU'LL BURN

YOU SAY: The more you sweat, the more fat you'll burn.

I SAY: You've seen those people at the gym—sitting in the sauna all day, exercising in plastic sweat suits, or even worse, sitting in the sauna all day *while wearing* a plastic sweat suit. Why do they do it? Because more sweat equals more fat burn. *Right?* Wrong! Fat loss is about burning calories, and saunas or sweat suits do not increase the number of calories burned. Furthermore, people often mistakenly judge the intensity, and by extension the effectiveness, of their workout by how much they sweat.

Just think about it: If it were true that more sweat equated to more calories burned, wouldn't you just be able to skip exercise altogether and spend all your time baking in a sauna to lose weight?

Fact is, sweat is just one of the many methods your body uses to control your core temperature. Sweat does not directly correlate to the intensity of your workout. Instead, the amount of sweat you produce is merely a reflection of the temperature and humidity of the air around you.

In addition, you are always sweating whether or not you're aware of it. When the air is hot, your body sweats more in hopes that the water will evaporate in the warm air, cooling your skin. When the air is very humid, though, it's more difficult for sweat to just evaporate off the skin. That's why it collects on your skin and even starts to drip, making it look like you're having a really killer workout.

So while you might have heard that intense sweating helps you shed pounds, or even experienced this result for yourself, it's important to keep in mind that the weight lost through intense sweating is just plain water weight. And once you rehydrate with a few glasses of water, you'll just gain all the weight back. So much for that plan!

The Dark Side of Sports and Sweat

Since sweat works to control your body's core temperature, it's generally not a good idea to mess with it. Doing so can raise your body's temperature to dangerously high levels. This was starkly demonstrated in 1997 when the National Collegiate Athletic Association took the step to ban rubber sweat suits after three wrestlers died while using them in a high-heat environment to try to drop weight before a match.

Furthermore, ramping up sweat production can easily lead to dehydration, which is in turn counter-productive to fat burn, not to mention your overall health. Case in point, severe dehydration can bump up production of the stress hormone cortisol, while lowering your testosterone levels, ultimately compromising your body's ability to burn fat.

Staying Hydrated

When it comes to fitness, I tell folks that what you drink is a lot more important than how much you sweat. The Institute of Medicine's Food and Nutrition Board recommends a daily fluid intake of 91 ounces for women and 125 ounces (about 1 gallon) for men. As a general guideline, I also advise that 90 percent of your liquid intake be water to keep yourself properly hydrating so you can be at your best for performance.

It's also important to note that while sweat is composed mostly of

water, it also contains essential minerals like sodium an
These minerals play a key role in muscle contractio
conduction, so losing them during exercise can negat
performance.

That said, for the average person who hits the gym, water will
be enough and the best option to meet your hydration needs.
However, in the case of elite athletes who typically undergo more
prolonged and intense workouts, sports drinks infused with
minerals and electrolytes are sometimes used to help rehydrate and
replenish.

Smarter than Sweat

While sweating won't give you an accurate measure of how intensely
you're exercising or how much fat you're burning, there are other
safe and fairly accurate methods to measure your workout intensity
and gauge fat burn.

One such measure is the Rate of Perceived Exertion (RPE) scale,
which allows you to rate your workout on a personalized scale of
1 to 10. Since what is incredibly easy to you might be impossible to
someone else and vice versa, it's important to understand that this
method of measuring workout intensity is quite subjective.

Similarly, many trainers like to use the "talk test" to monitor (and
control) their clients' exercise intensity. The "talk test" is basically
your ability to comfortably maintain a conversation while you're
exercising.

Bottom line: Regardless of whether you attempt to use measures
like RPE or the talk test, remember that fat loss is about burning
calories, and techniques like plastic sweat suits and saunas that are
simply meant to overheat the body and make you sweat more will not
significantly increase the number of calories your body burns. They'll
just make you sweat a ton, and sweat doesn't have anything to do with
dropping body fat. Furthermore, saunas and plastic sweat suits can
be dangerous, since they pose risks like dehydration and overheating.
Remember, when all is said and done, true weight loss boils down to

calories in versus calories out. Sweat ain't got nothing to do with it! So if you want to lose fat (not just water weight), I'd suggest skipping the sweat suit and sauna and focusing more on getting your diet and and exercise protocol in check. exercise protocol in check.

MISTAKE 18

COFFEE AND CAFFEINE ARE BAD FOR YOU

YOU SAY: Coffee and caffeine are bad for you.

I SAY: We Americans love our coffee. In fact, according to the National Coffee Association, some 83 percent of Americans indulge in at least one cup every day. Despite this propensity towards the ritual cup of coffee, many of us are frequently trying to cut back on just how much coffee we drink. Generally, this is done under the assumption that coffee, and all the caffeine found therein, is bad for you.

It turns out though that coffee has many health benefits, and when consumed sensibly, coffee (or even straight up caffeine) can even be a powerful tool to help you reach your fitness goals.

Weight Loss Benefits

Coffee is actually an incredibly complex substance, containing hundreds of chemicals that all have different effects on the human body. Of course, the most famous of these chemicals is caffeine. A potent stimulant, caffeine acts directly on our central nervous system to cause a spike in levels of dopamine and adrenaline. Both of these hormones give you a jolt of energy and elevate mood, but the adrenaline effect specifically is most appealing because adrenaline release directly causes an increase in the metabolism of body fat. Moreover, since caffeine has a stimulant effect, it can also improve overall athletic performance. This applies to both physical and mental performance, so consuming caffeine before a workout can, in fact, help you to focus better, work harder, and subsequently burn more calories.

Caffeine also has a thermogenic effect. Thermogenesis is the production of heat in the body, which also causes an increase in calorie expenditure. This means that caffeine consumption leads to more calories burned over time. Mind you, this thermogenic effect of caffeine won't make you lose tons of weight on its own, but it's definitely something that can give you a bit of an advantage in the overall weight loss race.

Two other chemicals found in coffee worth mentioning are chlorogenic acid and quinides. Both of these substances have a positive impact on the way that our body responds to sugar and insulin, which will subsequently help to improve weight loss while also helping to prevent diabetes.

Last, but definitely not least, caffeine also has the added benefit of being an appetite suppressant. And as we all know, by limiting the desire to eat, you'll more likely to eat less and lose more weight.

General Health Benefits of Coffee

Truth be told, coffee and caffeine can do a lot more than help you lose weight.

Regular coffee consumption has long been known to protect against liver disease, though the reason for the benefit remains unclear. Regular coffee consumption has also been shown to protect against liver and endometrial cancers, type 2 diabetes, gout, Alzheimer's disease, Parkinson's disease and other forms of dementia and cognitive decline.

Potential Caffeine Concerns

It is true that there are certain health concerns associated with coffee and caffeine. The primary issue is due to the stimulant effects of caffeine, as well as how the stimulant effects interact with certain preexisting conditions. Generally speaking, if you have cardiovascular disease, or are at risk for cardiovascular disease, you should be careful about your coffee or caffeine intake. Similarly, if you have issues with anxiety or have been diagnosed with an anxiety disorder, you should be mindful of caffeine consumption since it could exacerbate your condition.

Keep It Black

When enjoyed regularly and in moderation, coffee can offer incredible health benefits. Now mind you, when I talk about the benefits of regular coffee consumption, I'm talking about consuming real, antioxidant-rich organic black coffee and those not those 20-ounce caramel-mocha blendaccinos from your local coffee shop.

Many coffee shops are famous for maximal sugar, minimal coffee-based beverages that all too often are so heavily sweetened and so full of fat that the potential good of any real coffee that was added will be completely undone.

Bottom line: When it comes to your regular cup of joe, go organic and black. Worst case scenario, if you just can't stomach black coffee, it's okay to add a little bit of sugar or milk to make it more palatable. But avoid artificial sweeteners or sugary creamers. Another way to make your coffee more palatable is to add a little coconut oil. Coconut oil has tons of health benefits (including the ability to stimulate fat metabolism), and coconut oil will also give your coffee a sweet, pleasant aroma and a smoother taste.

earlier, a few factors can influence BMR, including your age, body composition, and sex. And while it seems pretty obvious that BMR would vary greatly from person to person, research suggests however that the difference in BMR from person to person may not be as large as anticipated.

In fact, a review of the available literature performed by researchers at the University of Vermont placed the metabolisms of 68 percent of the population within a range of five to eight percent of the average and 96 percent of people within 10 to 16 percent.

To better illustrate what this means, let's assume that the average BMR is 2,000 calories per day. What this study ultimately found was that 68 percent of people have a BMR between 1,800 and 2,200. Furthermore, for the vast majority of people, 96 percent, their BMR ranges between 1,700 and 2,300 calories per day. Altogether, this data means that the overwhelming majority of people have very similar metabolisms. Even when comparing the fastest against the slowest metabolisms, at a difference of about 600 calories, this is still considering the extreme ends of the spectrum that definitely wouldn't apply to the average person.

Eating Junk But Not Gaining Weight

And now you're probably shouting: *But what about people who eat junk food all the time and never gain a pound?!*

Yes, some people do have naturally faster metabolisms than others have. Their bodies can burn more energy while at rest, and so it's easier for them to stay lean and harder for them to gain weight. Are these people freaks of nature? Usually not. What I've found with people who have faster metabolisms is that they tend to have very good or excellent body composition in terms of the ratio of lean muscle mass to body fat. Excellent body composition is something you'll commonly see in people who make a conscious effort to lift weights and strength train, rather than just do cardio.

Still, although you may have come across one or a handful of people that seem to have this miraculous ability to eat junk and never gain weight, the fact remains that the difference between the fastest and the slowest of metabolisms just isn't as profound as many people think.

Furthermore, even in the case of people who can *seem* to eat whatever they want and never gain weight, I can guarantee you that those people don't eat nearly as many calories as you might think. Remember, as long as you aren't taking in excess calories, you won't gain weight. Even if all your calories come from junk food. Remember the story of Professor Mark Haub, who lost 27 pounds on his infamous "Twinkie Diet"?

All this is just to say that it's physiologically impossible for anyone to be able to lose weight while eating tons of excess calories every single day. That's just not how our bodies work. Weight loss, regardless of how difficult it may seem for some people, is simply about creating a caloric deficit while also maintaining insulin regulation.

Bottom line: If you've had difficulty losing weight, I'd strongly advise that you start taking a closer and more scrutinizing look at your nutritional protocol and your exercise program. The culprit behind your "slow metabolism" is most likely lurking there. As far as tools you could use, I'm a staunch advocate of keeping food diaries and workout calendars. There are tons of phone apps that can calculate your BMR and TDEE while allowing you to track the calories you take in from food and burn with exercise. You may also want to consider consulting a nutritionist to talk about healthy food changes you can make. Last but not least, if you still think you have slow metabolism, your doctor can run tests to check for conditions that can cause problems with metabolism, such as hypothyroidism and polycystic ovary syndrome (PCOS).

MISTAKE 20
SWITCHING TO DIET SODA WILL HELP YOU LOSE WEIGHT

YOU SAY: Switching to diet soda will help you lose weight.

I SAY: It's pretty much common knowledge these days that soda is bad for you. From the gobs of sugar to the preservatives to the artificial colorings and additives, these sweet bubbling beverages have been under fire in recent years due to their link with an increased risk of obesity and diabetes.

So in an effort to maintain their health, while also having the best of both worlds, many people have made the switch to diet soda. Many of the diet soda alternatives promised all the great taste, with zero calories and no sugar. So of course, for many people it seemed like a no-brainer to jump on the diet soda bandwagon.

Unfortunately, it turns out that diet sodas are in fact, doing much more harm than good.

Safe But Not Necessarily Healthy

Before they can proudly label their diet products as "zero calorie," food manufacturers must do a bit of creative engineering to their product. First, regular sugar has to be taken out of the formulary. But no sugar would leave soda flat and without its fizzle. So enter artificial sweeteners and other sugar substitutes.

In fact, there's a huge selection of calorie-free sugar substitutes for soda companies to choose from when formulating their diet soda product line, which is great for them. For the consumer though, many calorie-free sugar substitutes come with significant drawbacks in regards to health.

Most diet sodas are sweetened with at least one of these sugar substitutes: acesulfame potassium (marketed under the brand names Sunett and Sweet One), aspartame (Equal, NutraSweet), or sucralose (Splenda).

All of these sugar substitutes are FDA-approved and are therefore considered "safe" for human consumption. Notice I used the word "safe" and not "healthy." Technically speaking, just because a food item is deemed "safe" by the FDA does not make it a healthy addition to your diet. This mere fact has sent up numerous red flags all throughout the health community regarding the use of artificial sweeteners. Frustratingly though, the research is conflicting and mixed, and despite an ever-growing mass of laboratory studies in both humans and animals, we still don't have any conclusive ruling on the safety of all these products. Some studies show no link between artificial sweeteners and disease, while others demonstrate an increased risk of cancer, thyroid problems, tumors and even weight gain.

That's right: Some research suggests that diet sodas can actually make you *gain weight.*

Moreover, in a few cases, certain sugar substitutes were conclusively found to be harmful to humans and thus had to be removed from foods. For example, early on in the era of artificial sweeteners, a substance called cyclamate emerged. After a series of studies linked both cyclamate and saccharin to an increased risk of bladder cancer in rats, the FDA moved to ban cyclamate in 1969.

Another common sugar substitute you may have heard of with

possible health risks is aspartame. Though aspartame is FDA-approved and used in foods, studies have linked aspartame to lymphoma and leukemia in rats at very high doses (eight to 2,083 cans of diet soda daily). So while it is true that aspartame and other sweeteners, including acesulfame potassium, sucralose, and neotame, are still considered safe for human consumption by the FDA, it's still got to make you wonder—is diet soda really worth the risk to your health?

Dieting But Still Getting Fat

Sugar has many very interesting, and sometimes surprising, effects on the human brain. One example is the way that sugar affects appetite.

The natural course of things is that when you eat something sweet, that sweetness will trigger a chemical reaction that informs your brain that you just ate a food that's packed with calories. As a result, your brain works to suppress feelings of hunger so that you don't overeat.

However, some animal studies suggest that artificial sweeteners somehow disrupt this brain-appetite interaction so that our brain's ability to estimate caloric intake is thrown off. And in a study conducted at Purdue University's Ingestive Behavior Research Center, it was found that when rats were fed "no calorie" artificial sweeteners they ended up eating significantly more than those that just ate plain old table sugar, which ultimately led to a higher rate of obesity in the artificial sweetener rats.

Although the exact mechanism at work here isn't fully understood, the researchers theorized that the artificial sweeteners made the rats' brains think that they had just eaten a ton of calories. But when those calories didn't actually come and the brain didn't have as much fuel as it anticipated, the whole metabolic system went haywire. To try to recuperate those "missing" calories, the rats were overcome with an intense need to eat more. Interestingly enough, a similar effect on appetite has been noted in humans who consume artificial sweeteners too.

Zero Calories versus Calorie Free

Truth is, the FDA does allow manufacturers certain loopholes when it comes to food labels. Unfortunately, these loopholes are rarely ever in the best interest of the consumer.

So while you may opt for a diet soda because it promises you the same great taste with zero calories, you should keep in mind that apart from all the potential health risks just discussed, these "zero calorie" claims could be a half-truth. Put more plainly, that zero-calorie soda you've come to love could actually contain calories.

This fact may come as surprise, but according to FDA standards, food companies can get away with labeling a product as "calorie free" if it has fewer than five calories per serving. And while five calories might not sound like much, it can add up to quite a bit if you're downing several cans a day, a week, or a year.

Furthermore, when it comes to "low-calorie" labels, as long as the soda has between 30 and 40 calories per serving it can bear the "low-calorie" stamp. And the situation gets even worse if that zero-calorie soda is sweetened with aspartame, because your body does in fact break down this sweetener into methanol and amino acids, both of which generate calories once they enter your system. Of course, it is a fairly low number of calories. But once again, those calories do add up.

All Fizzled Out

The cold hard fact is that diet soda is no "healthier" than regular soda. Furthermore, diet soda isn't a better alternative for weight loss as seen from the effect it can have on appetite. So survey says: Dropping soda (regular or diet) from the typical foods you eat will go a long way towards improving your health.

And believe you me, I know soda can be difficult to give up. Personally, I was never a diet soda drinker, but I loved ginger ale. At one point several years ago, I was downing roughly one to two cans of ginger ale a day. Then I learned what soda was actually doing to my body and I quit cold turkey, which is the same advice I'd give others. I recommend quitting cold turkey and learning to get your "fizz fix" from healthier sources like flavored sparkling or regular sparkling water. For example, when I get a need for fizz, I love mixing ice-cold sparkling water with a few tablespoons of all-natural juice from Whole Foods, or I'll lightly sweeten my sparkling water with fresh squeezed fruit. This way, I can get my fizz, plus a few antioxidants and vitamins, without the potentially harmful chemicals that could make me sick or fat.

Is This The End?

Nope! This is just the beginning of your fitness journey—your journey to a slimmer, stronger and sexier you! Take all the wisdom contained in this book, go forth and prosper. I believe in you. Trust in yourself. You got this!

And don't forget to share the health and fitness gospel among your friends and family. Sharing is caring! So please recommend this book to anyone and everyone you think it would benefit. Also, please take a quick minute to leave a review on Amazon, or wherever you purchased my book. I've thoroughly enjoyed writing this book and sharing the information within, and I (as well as others) would definitely like to know your thoughts on my book.

Last, but definitely not least, be sure to keep a look out for more books to come, specifically *And That's Why You're Fat: Health & Fitness Mistakes to Stop Making, Volume 2* and beyond!

—Doc

About the Author

DR. PHOENYX AUSTIN is a Sports Medicine Physician, #1 Bestselling Author and Certified Trainer. Find her at DrPhoenyx.com.

Fitness Terms Everyone Should Know

Do you speak *gym*?

For some people, joining a gym can be pretty scary. It's almost like going to another country where everyone speaks a different language using words and phrases you've never heard before. And as if just the experience of joining a gym with all those hard bodies walking around wasn't intimidating enough, now you have to speak to people and pretend you know what other more seasoned gym folk are talking about.

If you're a total fitness newbie, gym-speak can get over your head at times. Sometimes I'll even meet newbies that will actually exclude themselves from certain areas of the gym, or will even avoid the gym at certain heavy-traffic times because they feel uncomfortable about not knowing gym slang or just basic fitness terms. That's why I thought it would be helpful to add this section to my book.

Below you'll find the most basic of fitness terms that everyone should know. Think of this as a crash course in "gym speak." Take a moment to read through and familiarize yourself with the lingo. And fret not, learning gym speak isn't difficult at all. Thankfully, there are only a few words you need to learn before you'll feel like a full-fledged "gym rat." Plus, learning the lingo will not only help you feel more comfortable among your fellow gym goers, but will also help you learn how to maximize your workouts.

EXERCISE AND GYM EQUIPMENT LINGO

Bar/Barbell: Used in strength training. A long straight bar (typically 45 pounds) to which weight plates can be affixed. Used traditionally for squats and bench presses.

Cables: A cable exercise apparatus typically comprises some type of handle, like a rope or

bar, attached to a pulley via a cable, which is then attached to some kind of stack of weights. By using the combination of handle, pulley, and cable, you can manipulate large amounts of weight and move in many different ranges of motion that would be difficult or impossible with a barbell or dumbbell.

Cardio: Short for cardiovascular exercise. Normally refers to workouts that get your heart rate elevated (i.e., treadmill, elliptical, stationary bike, swimming, aerobics class, and so forth). Cardiovascular exercise is designed primarily to work the heart and lungs.

Circuit training: A workout technique in which an individual performs a series of different exercises that are performed back to back with little to no rest in between. Circuit training helps to promote both muscle gain and cardiovascular health.

Collar: This is the attachment that secures the plate weights on a barbell or curl bar so the weight doesn't slip off.

Curl Bar: This curved bar, known as the EZ Curl or preacher curl bar, is typically used for biceps curls and normally weighs 25 pounds.

DOMS: Delayed-onset muscle soreness is the pain and stiffness felt in muscles several hours to days after unaccustomed or strenuous exercise. The soreness is felt most strongly 24 to 72 hours after the exercise. To treat DOMS, increase blood flow to the muscle with low-intensity work, massage or hot baths. Increased water and protein intake can also help repair muscles. Staying still can make DOMS worse.

Dumbbell: Used in strength training. Dumbbells typically comprise a handle in between two weights. They can be used individually, or you can use two at the same time (one in each hand). Dumbbells can be adjustable, meaning you can add resistance by attaching more weight to the dumbbell, or they can be fixed, meaning that you can't change the weight. Dumbbells are highly versatile and can be used for a wide range of exercises. You'll typically find them stored on a sturdy shelf called a "rack" or "dumbbell rack."

Failure: The point at which you cannot do one more rep. Failure simply means that you reached the point of physical exhaustion, which is often sought after in training protocols designed to build muscle.

Free weights: Standalone weights that aren't attached to some kind of pulley or machine. This term covers barbells, dumbbells, weight plates, medicine balls, kettlebells or anything else you can grab and do a variety of exercises with. Free weight exercises require more balance and engage more muscles than working out on universal machines. Free weights are good to include in a strength-training program because they are more challenging to use, train many stabilizing and balancing muscles, and offer a gym goer more versatility.

Get in/Work in: If you are asked by someone if they can "get in" or "work in," this means he or she would like to share a piece of equipment at the gym with you, perhaps by alternating sets on an exercise machine or using dumbbells that you're doing sets with.

High-intensity interval training (HIIT): High-intensity interval training is a form of interval training. The exercise strategy alternates periods of short, intense exercise with less intense recovery periods. See also Intervals.

Intervals: Intervals, or interval training, are a very effective technique that involves cycling between varying levels of intensity during cardiovascular exercise. For example, a 15-minute interval training protocol on the treadmill might comprise walking for 90 seconds, sprinting for 60 seconds, and then repeating the pattern. Intervals burn more calories and fat than running at a steady pace.

Max: See One-rep max.

Maximum heart rate: 220 minus your age. This number is frequently used when determining your appropriate training zone.

Negatives: Negative training is when the muscle lengthens during an exercise, also called an eccentric contraction. For instance, on a biceps curl, the negative movement is when you are bringing the weight back down. Concentric contraction is what we think of when we flex our muscle, or shorten the muscle (like the beginning of a biceps curl). The negative movement is believed to be a crucial part of muscle development.

One-rep max/Max: The maximum amount of weight one can lift in a single repetition.

Plates: Standalone weights of various increments that go on each end of a barbell or adjustable dumbbell. In America, plates typically weight 45, 35, 25, 10, 5 or 2.5 pounds, while most international plates are 25, 20, 17, 10, 5, 2.5, 2, or 1 kilogram.

PR or PB: Short for "personal record" or "personal best," these terms are used to describe a new personal achievement, such as running 3 miles in 20 minutes, or being able to bench press 200 pounds.

Pyramiding: Doing sets of downward or upward scaling of reps or weight. For example, pyramiding upward would be lifting one set of 60-pound weights, then lifting one set of 70-pound weights, then lifting one set of 80-pound weights.

Recovery: Refers to rest between exercises. When you perform an exercise, you'll eventually get to the point where you need a specified number of seconds or minutes to rest or go easy. That is referred to as your "recovery" period, and it typically varies from 30 seconds up to several minutes. Short recovery is best for fat burn and conditioning; long recovery is best for power lifting and bulking.

Rep: Short for repetition. Refers to one complete movement of one exercise (for example, a single push up).

Resistance training: See Strength training.

Set: A set is a group of repetitions. Typically, you will perform 2 to 8 or more sets for any given exercise (that is, one set of 8 reps). For example, if you are trying to get a toned butt, you might perform 5 sets of 12 reps of a reverse lunge exercise.

Spin: A form of cycling that is performed on a special bike called a Spin bike, usually occurring in a class setting. Typically, Spin bikes have a wheel called a "flywheel" that provides the resistance, so they're a bit different from a regular stationary bicycle.

Spot: When someone assists another person with an exercise. For example, "Can you spot me?" or, "I need a spotter."

Stack: On a weightlifting machine or cable apparatus, the resistance is provided by a stack, which is usually several rectangular-shaped plates that are stacked on top of one another. Resistance can be selected by using a pin that can be placed at a chosen place in the stack. Interestingly, a stack can also refer to taking several nutritional supplements at once.

Strength training/Resistance training: Any type of training that builds muscle by working against a form of resistance, usually weights, machines or resistance bands.

Super set: Refers to a combination of complimentary exercises done back to back in one "super set" with little to no rest in between each exercise. For instance, "I did a super set of shoulder presses and lateral raises."

Tabata training: Tabata training is a highly effective style of interval training that entails doing an exercise for 20 seconds of work and 10 seconds of rest for 8 rounds, totaling 4 minutes.

Tempo: Many workout books, magazines, or programs now indicate tempo, which simply refers to the speed at which you lift. For example, if you take 3 seconds to lift a weight, hold the weight for 1 second at the top of the movement, then take 2 seconds to lower the weight, the tempo would be 3:1:2.

Universal machines: Refers to weight machines where you can easily select a weight by inserting a pin in the weight stack. Universal machines can be used by pretty much anyone and are typically used when exercisers want to isolate a very specific muscle or body part for strength training.

Work in: See Get in.

ANATOMY AND BODY LINGO

Basal metabolic rate (BMR): Refers to the amount of calories you burn at rest.

Bi's: Biceps (the front part of the upper arm). People often use language like "bi's and tri's" as shorthand when talking about the body parts they trained.

Bulk/Bulking/Bulking up: Slang for adding muscle mass to one's body through strength training and nutrition.

Core: Refers to the conglomeration of "stabilizer" muscles that comprise your lower back, mid-back, abdominals and obliques. Your core is also sometimes called your "trunk."

Cut/Cutting/Cutting up: Slang term for decreasing the amount of body fat on one's body to better showcase musculature.

Definition: Low body fat coupled with developed musculature. Also called ripped, cut, or shredded.

Delts: Shoulders. You can work the front, middle and rear delts.

Glutes: Short for gluteus maximus, also known as buttocks, the largest muscles in the body. A much more sophisticated way to say "butt."

Hams: Hamstrings (back of the thighs). Also playfully called "hammies."

Jacked: Refers to a guy or girl who has a lot of muscle. For example, "That dude is jacked!"

Juice: A slang term for steroids (for example, "I think he's juicing...."). If you hear someone say they are on "juice," they aren't talking about juicing fruits and vegetables, they're talking about steroids.

Lats: Short for latissimus dorsi (back).

Lean body mass: The mass of your body minus the amount of fat, or just the amount of muscle you have. There are a number of equations and methods for calculating or determining lean body mass.

Pecs: Short for pectorals. This slang term refers to a person's chest muscles.

Pump: This is when your muscle is so full of glycogen and water from training that it will actually feel like it has been pumped up like a bicycle tire. It will feel tight to the touch and temporarily look swollen (in a good way).

Quads: Quadriceps (front of the thighs).

Ripped: Someone is ripped when they have very low body fat, and muscle separation is visible and defined. For example, "That dude is ripped!"

Traps: Short for trapezius muscles, which span across the neck, shoulders and upper back. Traps are the muscles you typically think of when you ask someone to rub your shoulders.

Tri's: Triceps (the back part of the upper arm). This is the part women hate to jiggle when they wave.

Selected References

2. Eat many small meals a day to boost metabolism

Bellisle, F., R. McDevitt, and A. M. Prentice. "Meal Frequency and Energy Balance." *The British Journal of Nutrition* 77 Suppl. 1 (1997): S57-S70. Print.

Cameron, J. D., M. J. Cyr, and E. Doucet. "Increased Meal Frequency Does Not Promote Greater Weight Loss in Subjects Who Were Prescribed an 8-Week Equi-Energetic Energy-Restricted Diet." *British Journal of Nutrition* 103.8 (2010): 1098-101. Print.

Leidy, Heather J. "The Effects of Consuming Frequent, Higher Protein Meals on Appetite and Satiety During Weight Loss in Overweight/ Obese Men." *Obesity (Silver Spring, Md.)* 19.4 (2011): 818-24. Print.

Leidy, Heather J., et al. "The Influence of Higher Protein Intake and Greater Eating Frequency on Appetite Control in Overweight and Obese Men." *Obesity (Silver Spring, Md.)* 18.9 (2010): 1725-32. Print.

LeSauter, Joseph, et al. "Stomach Ghrelin-Secreting Cells as Food-Entrainable Circadian Clocks." *Proceedings of the National Academy of Sciences* 106.32 (2009): 13582-87. Print.

3. Work your abs more to get rid of belly fat

Achten, Juul, and Asker E. Jeukendrup. "Optimizing Fat Oxidation through Exercise and Diet." *Nutrition (Burbank, Los Angeles County, Calif.)* 20.7-8 (2004): 716-27. Print.

Deldicque, Louise, et al. "Increased P70s6k Phosphorylation During Intake of a Protein-Carbohydrate Drink Following Resistance Exercise in the Fasted State." *European Journal of Applied Physiology* 108.4 (2010): 791-800. Print.

Derave, Wim, et al. "Effects of Post-Absorptive and Postprandial Exercise on Glucoregulation in Metabolic Syndrome." *Obesity (Silver Spring, Md.)* 15.3 (2007): 704-11. Print.

Kraemer, W. J., et al. "Acute Hormonal Responses to a Single Bout of Heavy Resistance Exercise in Trained Power Lifters and Untrained Men." *Canadian Journal of Applied Physiology = Revue Canadienne De Physiologie Appliquée* 24.6 (1999): 524-37. Print.

Maki, Kevin C., et al. "Green Tea Catechin Consumption Enhances Exercise-Induced Abdominal Fat Loss in Overweight and Obese Adults." *The Journal of Nutrition* 139.2 (2009): 264-70. Print.

Newsholme, E. A., and G. Dimitriadis. "Integration of Biochemical and Physiologic Effects of Insulin on Glucose Metabolism." *Experimental and Clinical Endocrinology & Diabetes: Official Journal, German Society Of Endocrinology [and] German Diabetes Association* 109 Suppl. 2 (2001): S122-S34. Print.

Surina, D. M., et al. "Meal Composition Affects Postprandial Fatty Acid Oxidation." *The American Journal of Physiology* 264.6 Pt 2 (1993): R1065-R70. Print.

Venables, Michelle C., et al. "Green Tea Extract Ingestion, Fat Oxidation, and Glucose Tolerance in Healthy Humans." *The American Journal of Clinical Nutrition* 87.3 (2008): 778-84. Print.

Vispute, Sachin S., et al. "The Effect of Abdominal Exercise on Abdominal Fat." *The Journal of Strength and Conditioning Research (Lippincott Williams & Wilkins)* 25.9 (2011): 2559-64. Print.

4. Low-carb diets are too hard to stick to

Aude, Y. Wady, et al. "The National Cholesterol Education Program Diet Vs a Diet Lower in Carbohydrates and Higher in Protein and Monounsaturated Fat: A Randomized Trial." *Archives of Internal Medicine* 164.19 (2004): 2141-46. Print.

Brehm, Bonnie J., et al. "A Randomized Trial Comparing a Very Low Carbohydrate Diet and a Calorie-Restricted Low Fat Diet on Body Weight and Cardiovascular Risk Factors in Healthy Women." *The Journal of Clinical Endocrinology and Metabolism* 88.4 (2003): 1617-23. Print.

Brinkworth, Grant D., et al. "Long-Term Effects of a Very-Low-Carbohydrate Weight Loss Diet Compared with an Isocaloric Low-Fat Diet after 12 Mo." *The American Journal of Clinical Nutrition* 90.1 (2009): 23-32. Print.

Dyson, P. A., S. Beatty, and D. R. Matthews. "A Low-Carbohydrate Diet Is More Effective in Reducing Body Weight Than Healthy Eating in Both Diabetic and Non-Diabetic Subjects." *Diabetic Medicine: A Journal of the British Diabetic Association* 24.12 (2007): 1430-35. Print.

Foster, Gary D., et al. "A Randomized Trial of a Low-Carbohydrate Diet for Obesity." *The New England Journal of Medicine* 348.21 (2003): 2082-90. Print.

Gardner, C. D., et al. "Comparison of the Atkins, Zone, Ornish, and Learn Diets for Change in Weight and Related Risk Factors among Overweight Premenopausal Women. The A to Z Weight Loss Study: A Randomized Trial." *Journal of the American Medical Association* 297.9 (2007): 969-77. Print.

Halyburton, Angela K., et al. "Low- and High-Carbohydrate Weight-Loss Diets Have Similar Effects on Mood but Not Cognitive Performance." *The American Journal of Clinical Nutrition* 86.3 (2007): 580-87. Print.

Hernandez, Teri L., et al. "Lack of Suppression of Circulating Free Fatty Acids and Hypercholesterolemia During Weight Loss on a

High-Fat, Low-Carbohydrate Diet." *The American Journal of Clinical Nutrition* 91.3 (2010): 578-85. Print.

Hession, M., et al. "Systematic Review of Randomized Controlled Trials of Low-Carbohydrate Vs. Low-Fat/Low-Calorie Diets in the Management of Obesity and Its Comorbidities." *Obesity Reviews: An Official Journal of the International Association for the Study of Obesity* 10.1 (2009): 36-50. Print.

Keogh, Jennifer B., et al. "Effects of Weight Loss from a Very-Low-Carbohydrate Diet on Endothelial Function and Markers of Cardiovascular Disease Risk in Subjects with Abdominal Obesity." *The American Journal of Clinical Nutrition* 87.3 (2008): 567-76. Print.

Krebs, Nancy F., et al. "Efficacy and Safety of a High Protein, Low Carbohydrate Diet for Weight Loss in Severely Obese Adolescents." *The Journal of Pediatrics* 157.2 (2010): 252-58. Print.

McClernon, F. Joseph, et al. "The Effects of a Low-Carbohydrate Ketogenic Diet and a Low-Fat Diet on Mood, Hunger, and Other Self-Reported Symptoms." *Obesity* 15.1 (2007): 182-87. Print.

Meckling, Kelly A., Caitriona O'Sullivan, and Dayna Saari. "Comparison of a Low-Fat Diet to a Low-Carbohydrate Diet on Weight Loss, Body Composition, and Risk Factors for Diabetes and Cardiovascular Disease in Free-Living, Overweight Men and Women." *The Journal of Clinical Endocrinology and Metabolism* 89.6 (2004): 2717-23. Print.

Nickols-Richardson, Sharon M., et al. "Perceived Hunger Is Lower and Weight Loss Is Greater in Overweight Premenopausal Women Consuming a Low-Carbohydrate/High-Protein Vs High-Carbohydrate/Low-Fat Diet." *Journal of the American Dietetic Association* 105.9 (2005): 1433-37. Print.

Samaha, Frederick F., et al. "A Low-Carbohydrate as Compared with a Low-Fat Diet in Severe Obesity." *The New England Journal of Medicine* 348.21 (2003): 2074-81. Print.

Shai, Iris, et al. "Weight loss with a low-carbohydrate, Mediterranean, or low-fat diet." *New England Journal of Medicine* 359.3 (2008): 229-241. Print.

Sondike, Stephen B., Nancy Copperman, and Marc S. Jacobson. "Effects of a Low-Carbohydrate Diet on Weight Loss and Cardiovascular Risk Factor in Overweight Adolescents." *The Journal of Pediatrics* 142.3 (2003): 253-58. Print.

Tay, Jeannie, et al. "Metabolic Effects of Weight Loss on a Very-Low-Carbohydrate Diet Compared with an Isocaloric High-Carbohydrate Diet in Abdominally Obese Subjects." *Journal of the American College of Cardiology* 51.1 (2008): 59-67. Print.

Volek, Jeff S. "Comparison of Energy-Restricted Very Low-Carbohydrate and Low-Fat Diets on Weight Loss and Body Composition in Overweight Men and Women." *Nutrition & Metabolism* 1.1 (2004): 13-13. Print.

Volek, Jeff S., et al. "Carbohydrate Restriction Has a More Favorable Impact on the Metabolic Syndrome Than a Low Fat Diet." *Lipids* 44.4 (2009): 297-309. Print.

Westman, Eric C., et al. "Low-Carbohydrate Nutrition and Metabolism." *The American Journal of Clinical Nutrition* 86.2 (2007): 276-84. Print.

Yancy, William S., Jr., et al. "A Low-Carbohydrate, Ketogenic Diet Versus a Low-Fat Diet to Treat Obesity and Hyperlipidemia: A Randomized, Controlled Trial." *Annals of Internal Medicine* 140.10 (2004): 769-77. Print.

5. For faster fat loss, exercise as often as possible, for as long as possible

Ahmaidi, S., et al. "Effects of Active Recovery on Plasma Lactate and Anaerobic Power Following Repeated Intensive Exercise." *Medicine and Science in Sports and Exercise* 28.4 (1996): 450-56. Print.

Kreher, Jeffrey B., and Jennifer B. Schwartz. "Overtraining Syndrome:

A Practical Guide." *Sports Health* 4.2 (2012): 128-38. Print.

Kuoppasalmi, K., et al. "Plasma Cortisol, Androstenedione, Testosterone and Luteinizing Hormone in Running Exercise of Different Intensities." *Scandinavian Journal of Clinical and Laboratory Investigation* 40.5 (1980): 403-09. Print.

Micklewright, D P., R Beneke, V Gladwell, and M H. Sellens. 2002. "Blood Lactate Removal Using Combined Massage and Active Recovery". Medicine & Science in Sports & Exercise. 35 (Suppl. ement 1): S317.

Mohammad Reza, Safarinejad. "The Effects of Intensive, Long-Term Treadmill Running on Reproductive Hormones, Hypothalamus–Pituitary–Testis Axis, and Semen Quality: A Randomized Controlled Study." *Journal of Endocrinology* 200.3 (2009): 259-71. Print.

Suzuki, M., et al. "Effect of Incorporating Low Intensity Exercise into the Recovery Period after a Rugby Match." *British Journal of Sports Medicine* 38.4 (2004): 436-40. Print.

6. Eating fat will make you fat

Baba, N., E. F. Bracco, and S. A. Hashim. "Enhanced Thermogenesis and Diminished Deposition of Fat in Response to Overfeeding with Diet Containing Medium Chain Triglyceride." *The American Journal of Clinical Nutrition* 35.4 (1982): 678-82. Print.

Enig, Mary G. "Coconut: In Support of Good Health in the 21st Century - Part II." *Mercola.com*. Joseph Mercola, 28 July 2001. Web. 17 Dec. 2013.

Fife, Bruce. "Hypothyroidism and Virgin Coconut Oil." *Coconut Connections*. n.p., 2001. Web. 17 Dec. 2013.

Fushiki, T., et al. "Swimming Endurance Capacity of Mice Is Increased by Chronic Consumption of Medium-Chain Triglycerides." *The Journal of Nutrition* 125.3 (1995): 531-39. Print.

Groves, Barry. "The Cholesterol Myth: Part 1 - Introduction." *Second*

Opinions. Barry Groves, 18 Sept. 2000. Web. 17 Dec. 2013.

---. " The Cholesterol Myth: Part 2 - Dietary Fats and Heart Disease." *Second Opinions.* Barry Groves, 18 Sept. 2000. Web. 17 Dec. 2013.

Isaacs, C. E., and K. Schneidman. "Enveloped Viruses in Human and Bovine-Milk are Inactivated by Added Fatty-Acids (FAS) and Monoglycerides (MGS)." *FASEB Journal.* 5.5 (1991): Abstract 5325, p. A1288. Print.

Isaacs, C. E., et al. "Addition of Lipases to Infant Formulas Produces Antiviral and Antibacterial Activity." *Journal of Nutritional Biochemistry* 3.6 (1992): 304-08. Print.

Kaunitz, H, and C.S Dayrit. "Coconut Oil Consumption and Coronary Heart Disease." *Philippine Journal of Internal Medicine.* 30.3 (1999): 165-171. Print.

Malhotra, Aseem. "Observations: Saturated Fat Is Not the Major Issue." (2013). *BMJ.* BMJ Publishing Group Ltd., 22 Oct. 2013. Web. 17 Dec. 2013.

Matsumoto, M., et al. "Defaunation Effects of Medium-Chain Fatty Acids and Their Derivatives on Goat Rumen Protozoa." *Journal of General and Applied Microbiology* 37.5 (1991): 439-45. Print.

Prior, I. A., et al. "Cholesterol, Coconuts, and Diet on Polynesian Atolls: A Natural Experiment: The Pukapuka and Tokelau Island Studies." *The American Journal of Clinical Nutrition* 34.8 (1981): 1552-61. Print.

Siri-Tarino, Patty W., et al. "Meta-Analysis of Prospective Cohort Studies Evaluating the Association of Saturated Fat with Cardiovascular Disease." *The American Journal of Clinical Nutrition* 91.3 (2010): 535-46. Print.

St-Onge, M. P., and P. J. H. Jones. "Greater Rise in Fat Oxidation with Medium-Chain Triglyceride Consumption Relative to Long-Chain Triglyceride Is Associated with Lower Initial Body Weight and Greater Loss of Subcutaneous Adipose Tissue." *International Journal of Obesity and Related Metabolic Disorders: Journal of the*

International Association for the Study of Obesity 27.12 (2003): 1565-71. Print.

7. Women will get bulky from lifting heavy weights

Chen, B. B., et al. "Thigh Muscle Volume Predicted by Anthropometric Measurements and Correlated with Physical Function in the Older Adults." *The Journal of Nutrition, Health & Aging* 15.6 (2011): 433-38. Print.

Consitt, Leslie A., Jennifer L. Copeland, and Mark S. Tremblay. "Endogenous Anabolic Hormone Responses to Endurance Versus Resistance Exercise and Training in Women." *Sports Medicine (Auckland, N.Z.)* 32.1 (2002): 1-22. Print.

Fried, L. P., and J. M. Guralnik. "Disability in Older Adults: Evidence Regarding Significance, Etiology, and Risk." *Journal of the American Geriatrics Society* 45.1 (1997): 92-100. Print.

Muscaritoli, M., et al. "Consensus Definition of Sarcopenia, Cachexia and Pre-Cachexia: Joint Document Elaborated by Special Interest Groups (Sig) "Cachexia-Anorexia in Chronic Wasting Diseases" And "Nutrition in Geriatrics"." *Clinical Nutrition (Edinburgh, Scotland)* 29.2 (2010): 154-59. Print.

Phillips, Stuart M. "Resistance Exercise: Good for More than Just Grandma and Grandpa's Muscles." *Applied Physiology, Nutrition, and Metabolism = Physiologie Appliquée, Nutrition et Métabolisme* 32.6 (2007): 1198-205. Print.

Vandervoort, Anthony A. "Aging of the Human Neuromuscular System." *Muscle & Nerve* 25.1 (2002): 17-25. Print.

West, Daniel W. D., et al. "Sex-Based Comparisons of Myofibrillar Protein Synthesis after Resistance Exercise in the Fed State." *Journal of Applied Physiology (Bethesda, Md.: 1985)* 112.11 (2012): 1805-13. Print.

Wolfe, Robert R. "The Underappreciated Role of Muscle in Health and Disease." *The American Journal of Clinical Nutrition* 84.3 (2006): 475-82. Print.

8. Fruit juice and fruit smoothies are healthy

"Juicing." American Cancer Society, n.d. Web. 17 Dec. 2013.

Catteau, C., et al. "Consumption of Fruit Juices and Fruit Drinks: Impact on the Health of Children and Teenagers, the Dentist's Point of View." *Archives De Pédiatrie: Organe Officiel De La Société Française De Pédiatrie* 19.2 (2012): 118-24. Print.

Palmer, J. R., et al. "Sugar-Sweetened Beverages and Incidence of Type 2 Diabetes Mellitus in African American Women." *Archives of Internal Medicine* 168 (2008): 1487-92. Print.

10. All calories are created equal

Park, Madison. "Twinkie Diet Helps Nutrition Professor Lose 27 Pounds." *CNNHealth*. Cable News Network, 8 Nov. 2010. Web. 17 Dec. 2013.

Weigle, David S., et al. "A High-Protein Diet Induces Sustained Reductions in Appetite, Ad Libitum Caloric Intake, and Body Weight Despite Compensatory Changes in Diurnal Plasma Leptin and Ghrelin Concentrations." *The American Journal of Clinical Nutrition* 82.1 (2005): 41-48. Print.

11. You should always stretch before exercise

Cramer, Joel T., et al. "An Acute Bout of Static Stretching Does Not Affect Maximal Eccentric Isokinetic Peak Torque, the Joint Angle at Peak Torque, Mean Power, Electromyography, or Mechanomyography." *The Journal of Orthopaedic and Sports Physical Therapy* 37.3 (2007): 130-39. Print.

Dawson, B., et al. "Effects of Immediate Post-Game Recovery Procedures on Muscle Soreness, Power and Flexibility Levels over the Next 48 Hours." *Journal of Science and Medicine in Sport / Sports Medicine Australia* 8.2 (2005): 210-21. Print.

Fletcher, Iain M., and Bethan Jones. "The Effect of Different Warm-up Stretch Protocols on 20 Meter Sprint Performance in Trained Rugby Union Players." *The Journal of Strength and Conditioning Research / National Strength and Conditioning Association* 18.4 (2004): 885-88. Print.

Fowles, J. R., D. G. Sale, and J. D. Macdougall. "Reduced Strength after Passive Stretch of the Human Plantarflexors." *Journal of Applied Physiology (Bethesda, Md.: 1985)* 89.3 (2000): 1179-88. Print.

Herbert, Robert D., et al. "Stretching to Prevent or Reduce Muscle Soreness after Exercise." *The Cochrane Database of Systematic Reviews* 7 (2011): CD004577. Print.

Herman, Katherine, et al. "The Effectiveness of Neuromuscular Warm-up Strategies, That Require No Additional Equipment, for Preventing Lower Limb Injuries During Sports Participation: A Systematic Review." *BMC Medicine* 10 (2012): 75-75. Print.

Herman, Sonja L., and Derek T. Smith. "Four-Week Dynamic Stretching Warm-up Intervention Elicits Longer-Term Performance Benefits." *The Journal of Strength and Conditioning Research / National Strength and Conditioning Association* 22.4 (2008): 1286-97. Print.

Hough, Paul A., et al. "Effects of Dynamic and Static Stretching on Vertical Jump Performance and Electromyographic Activity." *The Journal of Strength and Conditioning Research / National Strength and Conditioning Association* 23.2 (2009): 507-12. Print.

Kay, Anthony D., and Anthony J. Blazevich. "Effect of Acute Static Stretch on Maximal Muscle Performance: A Systematic Review." *Medicine and Science in Sports and Exercise* 44.1 (2012): 154-64. Print.

Kistler, Brandon M., et al. "The Acute Effects of Static Stretching on the Sprint Performance of Collegiate Men in the 60- and 100-M Dash after a Dynamic Warm-Up." *The Journal of Strength and Conditioning Research / National Strength and Conditioning Association* 24.9 (2010): 2280-84. Print.

La Torre, Antonio, et al. "Acute Effects of Static Stretching on Squat Jump Performance at Different Knee Starting Angles." *The Journal of Strength and Conditioning Research / National Strength and Conditioning Association* 24.3 (2010): 687-94. Print.

Lawrence, Hart. "Effect of Stretching on Sport Injury Risk: A Review." *Clinical Journal of Sport Medicine* 15.2 (2005): 113-13. Print.

Macpherson, P. C., M. A. Schork, and J. A. Faulkner. "Contraction-Induced Injury to Single Fiber Segments from Fast and Slow Muscles of Rats by Single Stretches." *The American Journal of Physiology* 271.5 Pt 1 (1996): C1438-C46. Print.

Moore, Marjorie Ann, and Robert S. Hutton. An electromyographic investigation of muscle stretching techniques. MS thesis. University of Washington, 1979.

Shrier, I. "Stretching before Exercise Does Not Reduce the Risk of Local Muscle Injury: A Critical Review of the Clinical and Basic Science Literature." *Clinical Journal of Sport Medicine: Official Journal of the Canadian Academy of Sport Medicine* 9.4 (1999): 221-27. Print.

---. "Stretching before Exercise: An Evidence Based Approach." *British Journal of Sports Medicine* 34.5 (2000): 324-25. Print.

Thacker, Stephen B., et al. "The Impact of Stretching on Sports Injury Risk: A Systematic Review of the Literature." *Medicine and Science in Sports and Exercise* 36.3 (2004): 371-78. Print.

Winchester, Jason B., et al. "Static Stretching Impairs Sprint Performance in Collegiate Track and Field Athletes." *The Journal of Strength and Conditioning Research (Lippincott Williams & Wilkins)* 22.1 (2008): 13-18. Print.

12. Fasting kills metabolism and puts your body in starvation mode

Mansell, P. I., I. W. Fellows, and I. A. Macdonald. "Enhanced Thermogenic Response to Epinephrine after 48-H Starvation in Humans." *The American Journal of Physiology* 258.1 Pt 2 (1990): R87-R93. Print.

Nair, K. S., et al. "Leucine, Glucose, and Energy Metabolism after 3 Days of Fasting in Healthy Human Subjects." *The American Journal of Clinical Nutrition* 46.4 (1987): 557-62. Print.

Owen, O. E., et al. "Protein, Fat, and Carbohydrate Requirements During Starvation: Anaplerosis and Cataplerosis."*The American Journal of Clinical Nutrition* 68.1 (1998): 12-34. Print.

Varady, Krista A., and Marc K. Hellerstein. "Alternate-Day Fasting and Chronic Disease Prevention: A Review of Human and Animal Trials." *The American Journal of Clinical Nutrition* 86.1 (2007): 7-13. Print.

Zauner, C., et al. "Resting Energy Expenditure in Short-Term Starvation Is Increased as a Result of an Increase in Serum Norepinephrine." *The American Journal of Clinical Nutrition* 71.6 (2000): 1511-15. Print.

13. You can "spot reduce" body fat with specific exercises

Matthews, Jessica. "Fit Life: Why Is the Concept of Spot Reduction Considered a Myth?" 4 Sept. 2009. Web. 17 Dec. 2013.

Vispute, Sachin S., et al. "The Effect of Abdominal Exercise on Abdominal Fat." *The Journal of Strength and Conditioning Research* 25.9 (2011): 2559-64. Print.

14. Don't eat late at night if you want to lose weight

Bellisle, F., R. McDevitt, and A. M. Prentice. "Meal Frequency and Energy Balance." *British Journal of Nutrition* 77 (1997): S57-70. Print.

Keim, N. L., et al. "Weight Loss Is Greater with Consumption of Large Morning Meals and Fat-Free Mass Is Preserved with Large Evening Meals in Women on a Controlled Weight Reduction Regimen." *The Journal of Nutrition* 127.1 (1997): 75-82. Print.

15. When doing cardio, you want your heart rate in the "fat-burning zone"

Boutcher, Stephen H. "High-Intensity Intermittent Exercise and Fat Loss." *Journal of Obesity* 2011 (2011): 868305-05. Print.

Knab, Amy M, R A. Shanley, Karen Corbin, Fuxia Jin, Wei Sha, and David C. Nieman. "A 45-Minute Vigorous Exercise Bout Increases Metabolic Rate for 19 Hours." *Medicine and Science in Sports and Exercise* 43 (2011): 266.

Mougios, V., et al. "Does the Intensity of an Exercise Programme Modulate Body Composition Changes?" *International Journal of Sports Medicine* 27.3 (2006): 178-81. Print.

Treuth, M. S., G. R. Hunter, and M. Williams. "Effects of Exercise Intensity on 24-H Energy Expenditure and Substrate Oxidation." *Medicine and Science in Sports and Exercise* 28.9 (1996): 1138-43. Print.

17. The more you sweat the more fat you'll burn

Judelson, Daniel A., et al. "Effect of Hydration State on Resistance Exercise-Induced Endocrine Markers of Anabolism, Catabolism, and Metabolism." *Journal of Applied Physiology (Bethesda, Md.: 1985)* 105.3 (2008): 816-24. Print.

18. Coffee and caffeine are bad for you

Acheson, K. J., et al. "Caffeine and Coffee: Their Influence on Metabolic Rate and Substrate Utilization in Normal Weight and Obese Individuals." *The American Journal of Clinical Nutrition* 33.5 (1980): 989-97. Print.

Andersen, Lene Frost, et al. "Consumption of Coffee Is Associated with Reduced Risk of Death Attributed to Inflammatory and Cardiovascular Diseases in the Iowa Women's Health Study." *The American Journal of Clinical Nutrition* 83.5 (2006): 1039-46. Print.

Arab, Lenore. "Epidemiologic Evidence on Coffee and Cancer." *Nutrition & Cancer* 62.3 (2010): 271-83. Print.

Arendash, Gary W., and Cao Chuanhai. "Caffeine and Coffee as Therapeutics against Alzheimer's Disease." *Journal of Alzheimer's Disease* 20 (2010): 117-26. Print.

Astorino, Todd A., and Daniel W. Roberson. "Efficacy of Acute Caffeine Ingestion for Short-Term High-Intensity Exercise Performance: A Systematic Review." *The Journal of Strength and Conditioning Research / National Strength and Conditioning Association* 24.1 (2010): 257-65. Print.

Bruce, M., et al. "Anxiogenic Effects of Caffeine in Patients with Anxiety Disorders." *Archives of General Psychiatry* 49.11 (1992): 867-69. Print.

Costa, João, et al. "Caffeine Exposure and the Risk of Parkinson's Disease: A Systematic Review and Meta-Analysis of Observational Studies." *Journal of Alzheimer's Disease: JAD* 20 Suppl. 1 (2010): S221-S38. Print.

Gavrieli, A., et al. "The effect of different doses of caffeinated coffee on energy intake and appetite feelings of healthy male and female volunteers." *Proceedings of the Nutrition Society* 70.OCE6 (2011): E346.

Huxley, Rachel, et al. "Coffee, Decaffeinated Coffee, and Tea Consumption in Relation to Incident Type 2 Diabetes Mellitus: A Systematic Review with Meta-Analysis." *Archives of Internal Medicine* 169.22 (2009): 2053-63. Print.

Masterton, Gail Susan, and Peter C. Hayes. "Coffee and the Liver: A Potential Treatment for Liver Disease?"*European Journal of Gastroenterology & Hepatology* 22.11 (2010): 1277-83. Print.

Salazar-Martinez, Eduardo, et al. "Coffee Consumption and Risk for Type 2 Diabetes Mellitus." *Annals of Internal Medicine* 140.1 (2004): 1-8. Print.

Santos, Catarina, et al. "Caffeine Intake and Dementia: Systematic Review and Meta-Analysis." *Journal of Alzheimer's Disease* 20 (2010): 187-204. Print.

Shearer, Jane, et al. "Quinides of Roasted Coffee Enhance Insulin Action in Conscious Rats." *The Journal of Nutrition* 133.11 (2003): 3529-32. Print.

Singh, Jasvinder A., Supriya G. Reddy, and Joseph Kundukulam. "Risk Factors for Gout and Prevention: A Systematic Review of the Literature." *Current Opinion in Rheumatology* 23.2 (2011): 192-202. Print.

Van Dijk, Aimée E., et al. "Acute Effects of Decaffeinated Coffee and the Major Coffee Components Chlorogenic Acid and Trigonelline on Glucose Tolerance." *Diabetes Care* 32.6 (2009): 1023-25. Print.

19. I can't lose weight because my metabolism is slow

Donahoo, William T., James A. Levine, and Edward L. Melanson. "Variability in Energy Expenditure and Its Components." *Current Opinion in Clinical Nutrition and Metabolic Care* 7.6 (2004): 599-605. Print.

Park, Madison. "Twinkie Diet Helps Nutrition Professor Lose 27 Pounds." *CNNHealth*. Cable News Network, 8 Nov. 2010. Web. 17 Dec. 2013.

Tata, J. R., L. Ernster, and O. Lindberg. "Control of Basal Metabolic Rate by Thyroid Hormones and Cellular Function." *Nature* 193 (1962): 1058-60. Print.

20. Switching to diet soda will help you lose weight

Lim, Unhee, et al. "Consumption of Aspartame-Containing Beverages and Incidence of Hematopoietic and Brain Malignancies." *Cancer Epidemiology, Biomarkers & Prevention* 15.9 (2006): 1654-59. Print.

National Cancer Institute. "National Cancer Institute Factsheet: Artificial Sweeteners and Cancer." 5 Aug. 2009. Web. 17 Dec. 2013.

Soffritti, M., et al. "Aspartame Induces Lymphomas and Leukaemias in Rats." European Journal of Oncology 10.2 (2005): 107-16. Print.

Made in the USA
Lexington, KY
25 April 2014